Body
MASSAGE
THERAPY BASICS

Body

MASSAGE

THERAPY BASICS

Mo Rosser
● ● ● ● ● ● ●

Hodder & Stoughton

A MEMBER OF THE HODDER HEADLINE GROUP

Orders: please contact Bookpoint Ltd,
130 Milton Park, Abingdon,
Oxon OX14 4SB.

Telephone: (44) 01235 427720,
Fax: (44) 01235 400454. Lines are open from 9.00–6.00,
Monday to Saturday, with a 24 hour message answering service.
You can also order through our website www.hodderheadline.co.uk

British Library Cataloguing in Publication Data
A catalogue record for this title is available from the British Library

ISBN 0 340 81660 0

First Edition published 1996
Second Edition published 2004
Impression number   10 9 8 7 6 5 4 3 2
Year   2007 2006 2005 2004

Cover photo from: Doug Plummer/Photonica

Typeset by Charon Tec Pvt. Ltd, Chennai, India
Printed in Great Britain for Hodder & Stoughton Educational, a division of Hodder Headline,
338 Euston Road, London NW1 3BH by Martins the Printers, Berwick upon Tweed.

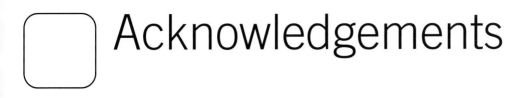

Acknowledgements

I am indebted to my friends and colleagues at the London College of Fashion for their encouragement and support during the preparation of this book.

I would like to thank my family for all their help and support; a special thanks to Greta Couldridge for her help, advice and support.

Finally my thanks to the following students for their time and patience while modelling for the photographs: Emma Avis, Lisa Barham, Nicola Christodulou and Georgina Vassili.

Mo Rosser

The publishers would like to thank the following individuals and institutions for permission to reproduce copyright material:

© Ronald Sheridan/Ancient Art & Architecture Collection Ltd: Figure 0.1; © The British Library, Or.6810,f.27v: Figure 0.2; © Andrew Brookes/Corbis: Figure 1.1; © Michael Keller/Corbis: Figure 3.1; © Carlton Professional: Figures 10.1, 10.2; © Dimitri Iundt/Corbis: Figure 11.1.

The commissioned photographs were taken by Susan Ford.

Every effort has been made to obtain necessary permission with reference to copyright material. The publishers apologise if inadvertently any sources remain unacknowledged and will be glad to make the necessary arrangements at the earliest opportunity.

Contents

Introduction

This book has been revised and updated to meet the new standards and requirements of the various awarding bodies. It will provide the student with a comprehensive introduction to massage and will also be of value to those already practising in this field. The broad-based information provided will guide the therapist towards safe and effective practice. For those wanting to progress further, additional information explaining some advanced massage techniques and the techniques of passive movements has been included, together with the rationale for their use.

Great emphasis is placed on the responsibility carried by every therapist to be well informed and to maintain the highest standards of safety and hygiene. Relevant information regarding the regulations and legal requirements is provided. The text will provide underpinning knowledge of anatomy and physiology, and will explain the application and the effects of massage on body systems and tissues. Guidance is also provided for dealing with, and caring for, each client on an individual basis. Contra-indications are carefully explained and advice given on the appropriate action to be taken.

The importance of consultation and accurate assessment is discussed, with guidance on meeting the needs of each client. Advice is given on planning effective treatments, selecting appropriate techniques and setting realistic targets.

Consideration is also given to the timing and costing of treatments, together with post-treatment observations and feedback.

Emphasis is placed throughout on high standards of client care and all the factors that will contribute to the success and effectiveness of the treatment.

Revision notes and questions are included among the text or at the end of each chapter, with model answers at the end of the book.

The aim of the book is to help the student become a caring, competent and successful practitioner. It will emphasise that the accomplished therapist will require an understanding of biological principles, an appreciation of the technique and effects of all massage manipulations, together with highly developed motor skills, sensitivity, integrity and dedication.

Massage forms an important part of all courses in beauty therapy, and also in the growing field of holistic and complementary therapies. Many techniques are combined with shiatsu, and acupressure routines, while the application of aromatic oils through massage is the basis of aromatherapy treatments.

Therapeutic techniques are once again recognised in mainstream medicine, for the relief of pain, improving the circulation and in general health care. Basic massage and other more advanced techniques are now carried out in hospitals, health centres, clinics etc, by therapists, nurses, and other health staff who have received training in these specialised areas. Athletes, sportspeople, dancers and actors include massage in their training schedules to aid recovery, promote relaxation and to prevent or treat soft tissue injuries. A qualification in massage offers numerous opportunities for employment in a variety of establishments such as beauty salons, health spas/clinics, leisure centres, sports complexes, and also in hair and beauty centres in hotels, large department stores and on board luxury cruise liners.

Massage continues to be practised throughout the world and we have much to learn from other cultures. It is hoped that this book will provide students with a sound foundation on which to build, explore and evaluate other techniques and theories. Expertise and excellence will develop through constant practice, self-assessment and evaluation of results. Massage offers an extremely rewarding and fulfilling career for those seeking a caring role in society.

Learning and assessment guidance

This book provides the basic information and direction for those interested in studying head and body massage treatments.

The material has been selected and organised to meet the requirements set by the various awarding bodies in line with National Standards. The text includes the main components, namely *underpinning knowledge, understanding* and *skill instruction.*

When you pursue this course of study and practice, you will acquire:

1 the underpinning knowledge and understanding to make you a safe and competent practitioner

2 the skills necessary to perform all the massage manipulations on the various parts of the body and on different types of client.

❖ *Learning* ❖

Skills learning

Learning how to massage is the same as learning any other skill, such as playing an instrument. You may find it difficult at the beginning but it will become easier with practice and experience. The more you practise, the faster you will improve. Watch carefully when manipulations are demonstrated by your tutor, then practise these yourself to develop the correct techniques immediately.

Before you start practising, learn the names of the main groups and the type of movement involved, e.g. those in the *effleurage* group are stroking movements; those in the *petrissage* group are kneading or pressure movements. Then learn the names of each manipulation and the movement involved.

Massage manipulations vary greatly in the dexterity required to perform them; some are very much easier than others.

Each time you practise a new manipulation try to break the movement down into small steps. Practise each step on a model until you are satisfied that you are performing them correctly, then link them together to perform the complete movement. The text has been organised to help you follow this step-by-step approach. Follow the technique section for every

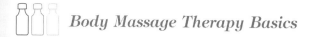

manipulation. Once you have mastered the movement you can then move on and concentrate on improving co-ordination of speed, depth and rhythm.

Remember that regular practice of hand exercises will improve strength and dexterity.

Knowledge and understanding

You will require background knowledge to be competent in your work and to be able to explain the effects and benefits of the treatment to your clients.

Health and safety legislation

You must understand the health, safety and welfare requirements related to your work. These will enable you to practise safely and protect yourself, colleagues and clients from harm. The relevant health, safety and welfare issues are discussed in the next chapter together with Local Authority regulations. These are legal requirements for all people in the workplace and are concerned with the hazards and risks in your place of work. They cover important emergency procedures such as fire drill and first aid.

They include safety issues related to equipment and practices, and stress the importance of high standards of hygiene, which must be practised at all times to prevent the spread of diseases; staff, clients and others must be protected from cross-infection and infestation. Hygiene relates to your own personal appearance and hygiene practices, e.g. clean overall, short nails, frequent bathing, hand washing before touching the client and after each treatment. It includes salon hygiene, e.g. clean boil-washed linen and towels for each client, prompt and safe disposal of waste into covered waste bins. It also covers client hygiene such as taking a shower before treatment, cleansing the areas to be massaged, checking and dealing with any contra-indications.

Communication

You must be able to communicate effectively and pleasantly with all types of people. You must recognise the importance of carrying out and recording a detailed client consultation and obtaining a signed consent form before starting the treatment. You must be able to create the right conditions and prepare the room and the client for treatment.

Anatomy and physiology

A knowledge of the structure and function of the body is necessary, as this will enable you to identify the structures you are working over and understand the effects produced on the body systems.

It will help you to learn this subject if you try to visualise the tissues underneath your hands as they move over a part when massaging.

Your hands are in contact with the skin: what is the skin composed of? Could you draw and label a section through the skin?

Under the skin is the subcutaneous layer: what is it made of?

Under this lie the muscles: can you name these muscles and give their action?

Under the muscles lie the bones connected at joints: can you name the bones and the joints?

In this book you will find the anatomy of each part immediately before the massage routine for that area, e.g. the anatomy of the leg is immediately before the leg massage routine. As you massage the leg, think of the structures underneath your hands and mentally answer the following:

➤ Name the bones and the joints that lie underneath.

➤ Name the muscles and note the fleshy parts, which can take heavier manipulations and are easier to knead, wring, pick up and roll than the more tendinous parts.

➤ Name the lymph nodes and their location.

Remember that arteries are deep, and blood flow through the arteries is governed by the contraction of the heart. You are not likely to affect this arterial blood flow with massage. Veins lie towards the surface, therefore massage will increase blood flow in the superficial veins.

Lymphatic vessels lie throughout the tissues and the flow of lymph will be increased by massage.

Revise the relevant anatomy both before and after the massage lesson. It becomes easier to remember when you relate it to practical work.

During assessment you may be required to give the name, position and action of certain superficial muscles.

You are required to know the parts and functions carried out by the body systems and how massage may affect them.

When you are studying the text, use the summaries, write your own notes on key points, ask yourself questions and answer them.

❖ **Assessment** ❖

◎ Any assessment is an opportunity for you to show how able you are. You will provide evidence of this ability to the assessor, who will judge your performance against the requirements of the awarding body.

◎ Throughout the course you will be required to provide various types of evidence, which the assessor will judge and say 'Yes this student is competent and capable of working to the National Standards'.

◎ Do not be apprehensive when you come to be assessed. Providing you have worked consistently you will have gained the skills and knowledge required to succeed. You may decide when you are ready to be assessed.

◎ Each assessment is your chance to demonstrate how good you are, and to provide evidence of your knowledge or skill.

◎ This book has been designed to help you achieve your goals.

◎ Ask your tutor or teaching centre for a copy of the unit you are studying. Do this at the beginning of the course. Read each section carefully. The unit will tell you exactly what you need to know. Do not be put off or be apprehensive as you read it; remember that you are going to acquire this knowledge one step at a time. Each awarding body will specify its own requirements but they must all work towards the same National Standards.

The Hairdressing and Beauty Industry Authority (HABIA) identifies the skill needs in these industries and sets the standards of competence, knowledge and understanding required to meet these needs. Units can be downloaded from the website of the awarding body; your college or tutor will have this information. The HABIA website is www.habia.org.

Remember, you are responsible for providing evidence of your competence; your tutor or assessor will help you by providing guidance and support. Make sure that you understand what is required of you.

If you know where you are going you are more able to help yourself get there.

Discuss the unit with your assessor, and develop and agree assessment plans. Make sure that you understand the procedure and what evidence is to be presented at each assessment.

You may have past experience and achievements that may count towards the competence for this unit. This is usually referred to as accreditation of prior learning. Remember to ask if past employment or training can be taken into account.

Before undertaking any assessment, the assessor must provide you with a list of criteria and the range statements. These will inform you of the knowledge and skill competences required to succeed.

The assessor should read through the criteria and range statements with you and offer support and advice. Make sure you understand everything that is said and ask for clarification if in doubt.

Your assessor will watch you working and will assess your performance against National Standards. You and the assessor will decide on the type of assessment and where the assessment is to take place. Evidence may be collected when you are treating a client in college or in the workplace. More evidence may be gathered through special tasks, e.g. projects or case studies. Your knowledge may be assessed by oral or written questions.

You may produce evidence in different ways:

◎ Being observed performing massage a specific number of times on different types of client. This will demonstrate that you have the necessary skills to carry out a full body massage including face and head, and that you can adapt the manipulations to suit the needs of different clients.

◎ You may be questioned by the assessor during or after the performance. Do not stop the massage when questioned unless told to do so. Learn and practise answering questions whilst massaging without losing rhythm.

◎ You may produce evidence of knowledge and understanding by writing assignments, projects or answering written questions.

Some suggestions for topics suitable for projects are:

a) Health and safety requirements: are these being upheld in your college or workplace? Information can be obtained from the Health and Safety Executive (HSE) at www.hse.gov.uk.

b) Lubricants used for massage, their advantages and disadvantages. Information on these products could be obtained from manufacturers, journals, magazines or exhibitions.

c) Adaptation of massage for different types of client and differing skin types. This could be supported by video evidence, photographs, record cards, letters, etc.

After every assessment you will be given feedback by your assessor. S/he will discuss your performance with you and tell you if you have been successful or unsuccessful. If you have been successful this will be recorded. If you have not been successful you will be offered further training. You have the right to appeal against an assessor's decision; your training centre will inform you of the procedure to follow should you wish to do so. You will find it helpful to keep your own written record of each piece of evidence as you provide it and an account of every practical assessment. Include the comments and advice of the assessor.

All the evidence you produce to demonstrate competence, knowledge and understanding is recorded and collected into a portfolio of evidence that is finally presented for certification.

Remember, to succeed you must:

➤ satisfy all evidence requirements

➤ meet all performance criteria

➤ include all aspects of the range

➤ meet all knowledge and understanding requirements.

Brief history of massage

After you have studied this chapter you will be able to:
1. explain how massage was used in ancient civilisations
2. explain the derivation of the word 'massage'
3. describe the development of massage from ancient to modern times
4. explain why massage became little used as a therapeutic treatment in hospitals
5. discuss the development of massage in the beauty and leisure industries.

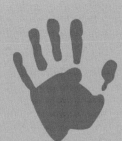

Massage has been practised throughout the centuries since the earliest civilisations. It has been used medically as a therapeutic healing treatment and also for invigorating, soothing and beautifying the body. Massage or rubbing is an instinctive act for relieving pain and discomfort, and for soothing and calming. The use of fats and aromatic oils for anointing and lubricating the body is referred to in the Bible and the Koran.

The word 'massage' has its origin in the Arabic word *mass* or *mass'h*, which means 'to press gently'. The Greek word *massage* means 'to knead' and the French word *masser* means 'to massage'.

Massage in ancient times

The earliest evidence of massage being used is found in the cave paintings of ancient cave dwellers. These wall drawings and paintings show people massaging each other. Various artefacts also found contain traces of fats and oils mixed with herbs. These indicate that lubricants may have been used, perhaps for healing, soothing or beautifying purposes.

As early as 3000 BC, the Chinese practised massage to cure ailments and improve general health. Records of this can be found in the British Museum. Ancient Chinese books record lists of massage movements with descriptions of their technique. One of these books, *The Cong Fau of Tao-Tse*, also contains lists of exercises and massage used to improve general health and well-being. The Chinese found that pressure techniques were very effective on specific points and they developed special techniques called *amma* (see Figure 0.1). This was the beginning of the development of acupressure and acupuncture.

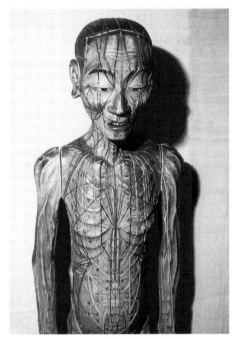

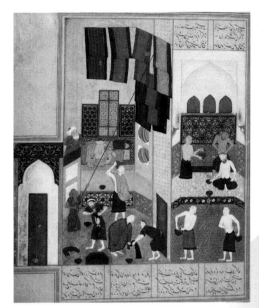

Figure 0.1 **An ancient Chinese acupuncture and massage study figure, showing treatment points.**

Figure 0.2 **This ancient Persian document shows bathing and massage in a Turkish bath.**

These massage techniques spread to Japan, where they were further developed. The Japanese used similar pressure techniques on specific points, which they called *tsubo*. This form of massage has been practised over the centuries; it has recently regained recognition and popularity and is now known as *shiatsu*. Many therapists have studied these techniques, which they combine with other forms of treatment for the benefit of their clients.

Records show that the Hindus practised massage as part of their hygiene routines. A sacred book called the *Ayur-Veda* (The Art of Life), which was written around 1800 BC, describes how shampooing and rubbing were used to reduce fatigue and promote well-being and cleanliness.

The Egyptians and Persians used massage for cosmetic as well as therapeutic effects (see Figure 0.2). They mixed fats, oils, herbs and resins for care of the skin and beautifying the body and face. Pots and jars containing these creams have been found in Egyptian tombs. Cleopatra is said to have bathed in milk and then to have been massaged with aromatic oils and creams by her handmaidens.

The practice of massage spread from the east into Europe, where it was well established by 500 BC.

Massage in classical Greece and Rome

The Greeks believed in the cultivation of a healthy mind and body, which is similar to the 'holistic approach' practised by many people today. Rituals of bathing, massage, exercise or dancing were practised by men and women. They encouraged the pursuit of physical fitness and organised regular sporting, gymnastic and athletic competitions. Massage was used before events to improve performance and after events to relieve fatigue and aid recovery. Gladiators and soldiers were massaged before battle to give vigour and promote fitness and health, and afterwards to aid recovery, healing and relaxation. Homer writes in the poem *The Odyssey* of Greek soldiers being rubbed with oils and anointed by beautiful women to aid their recovery and regain strength on return from battle.

Around 500 BC the Greek physician Herodicus used massage with oils and herbs to treat medical conditions and diseases. Hippocrates, who is now thought of as the father of medicine, was a pupil of Herodicus. He began to study the effects of massage on his patients. He concluded and recorded that 'hard rubbing binds, soft rubbing loosens, much rubbing causes parts to waste but moderate rubbing makes them grow'. Hippocrates also concluded that it was more beneficial to apply pressure in an upward direction, i.e. towards the heart, as we practise today. In Hippocrates' day, the function of the heart and the circulation of the blood were not known. It is therefore remarkable that he reached this conclusion only by observing the effect on the tissues of different strokes. With our knowledge of the heart and circulating blood we understand why pressure upwards is more beneficial: the condition of the tissues improves because deoxygenated blood and waste products are removed quickly as massage speeds up blood and lymph flow. Even without the benefit of this knowledge, Hippocrates taught his pupils that massage movements should be performed with pressure upwards to promote healing.

The Romans followed similar routines to the Greeks. They practised bathing, exercise and massage for health and social relaxation. Large private and public baths were built. These included water baths and steam rooms, gymnasium and massage areas. The baths were maintained at different temperatures and progress was made from cold to hot baths. Wealthy Romans would use these daily for cleansing, exercising, relaxing and socialising. Servants were always in attendance, with oils and creams to massage their masters when required. The Romans built similar baths in the countries that were conquered by their armies. Many such baths were built after the Roman conquest of Britain in 55 BC, and their ruins can be seen in Britain today in towns and cities such as Bath, Caerleon and St Albans. Massage techniques recorded from those times include manipulations known as squeezing, pinching or pummelling. They relate to the petrissage and percussion movements used today.

The Dark Ages to the Renaissance

Little is known about massage or health and beauty practices throughout the Dark and Middle Ages, i.e. from the decline of the Roman Empire around 500 AD until the Middle Ages around

1400 AD. Few records remain from those days of wars, strict religions, superstition and persecution. Little value was placed on education, the arts, physical health and fitness.

Following this period came the Renaissance (rebirth) in 1450 AD. Interest in the arts and sciences flourished and there was renewed interest in health practices. Once again we see massage advocated and practised for therapeutic purposes.

In the sixteenth century, the French surgeon Ambroise Paré (1517–90) promoted and developed the use of massage. He was the personal physician to four French kings. He is reputed to have successfully treated Mary Queen of Scots with massage. Paré graded massage into gentle, medium and vigorous. We use similar categories today, namely soothing or relaxing, general, and stimulating. Many other physicians copied his methods and massage was established medically.

The development of modern massage techniques

Modern massage techniques have evolved mainly from a system developed by a Swedish physiologist called Per Henrik Ling (1776–1839). He developed a system of passive and active exercises known as 'Swedish Remedial Gymnastics' and also a system of massage movements. Ling used the terms 'effleurage', 'petrissage', 'vibration', 'friction', 'rolling' and 'slapping'. Most of these terms are still used today, but some changes and modifications have been made in the groupings and names of manipulations.

Dr Johann Mezgner (1839–1909), a Dutch physician, developed massage for use in rehabilitation and used it successfully to treat many diseases and disorders. He adapted massage techniques in the light of his knowledge of anatomy and physiology. His theories, based on sound scientific principles, became accepted as medical practice and gained him many followers, particularly in Germany and America.

The work of Ling and Mezgner established massage as an effective therapeutic treatment. Techniques were taught in medical schools and the beneficial effects became widely recognised and accepted in the medical field. In England, the eminent surgeon John Grosvenor (1742–1823) used massage to treat joints. He recommended massage for the treatment of rheumatism, gout and stiffness of joints.

Nurses were encouraged to train and use massage for the treatment of patients, under the guidance of doctors. In 1894 a group of women founded the Society of Trained Masseuses. Rules and regulations for training and examinations for qualifying were established. These women raised standards and fought to establish massage therapy as a reputable profession.

Twentieth-century developments

During the First World War the demand for massage to treat the injured grew and many more massage therapists were trained. Membership of the Society of Trained Masseuses grew and in 1920 it amalgamated with the Institute of Massage and Remedial Exercise. In recognition of the valuable work contributed by its members during the war, a Royal Charter was granted and the title was changed to the Chartered Society of Massage and Medical Gymnastics. The title was changed again in 1943 and became the Chartered Society of Physiotherapy. In 1964 its members became state registered. This protected and gave status to those qualified therapists who were practising in clinics and hospitals, and made it impossible for those without a recognised qualification to practise in hospitals.

With the development of alternative electrical-based treatments, the use of massage to treat medical conditions declined. There was rapid growth in electrotherapy and eventually massage ceased to be part of physiotherapy training. It became little used as a therapeutic treatment in hospitals. There was, however, a continuing demand for massage in clinics, health farms, fitness and leisure centres.

In 1966 the City and Guilds of London Institute explored the possibility of establishing a course in beauty therapy to include massage. This course would provide thorough training, background knowledge and a recognised professional qualification that ensured a high standard of practice. In 1968 the first full-time course was offered in colleges of further education. The British Association of Beauty Therapists and Cosmetologists, the International Health and Beauty Council and other organisations also developed courses and offered certificates and diplomas. The growth in complementary medicine and the holistic approach to health has increased the demands for well-qualified practitioners, not only in massage but also in aromatherapy, reflexology, shiatsu etc. Courses are now validated by the Health and Beauty Therapy Training Board and therapists must meet the criteria of the National Council of Vocational Qualifications.

QUESTIONS

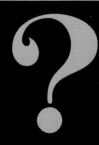

1. Outline the evidence which indicates that massage was practised by cave dwellers.
2. Name three languages from which the word 'massage' may have derived.
3. Explain briefly what is meant by the Chinese technique of acupuncture.
4. Describe briefly how the Greeks and Romans incorporated massage into their rituals.
5. Name the Greek physician who concluded that massage pressure should be applied in an upward direction.
6. Explain why little is known about massage in the Dark Ages.
7. Name three eminent doctors who promoted massage for healing purposes.
8. Explain why the reputation of massage grew during and after the First World War.
9. Name the examining body that established the first beauty therapy course in colleges of further and higher education.

Part A

Underpinning knowledge

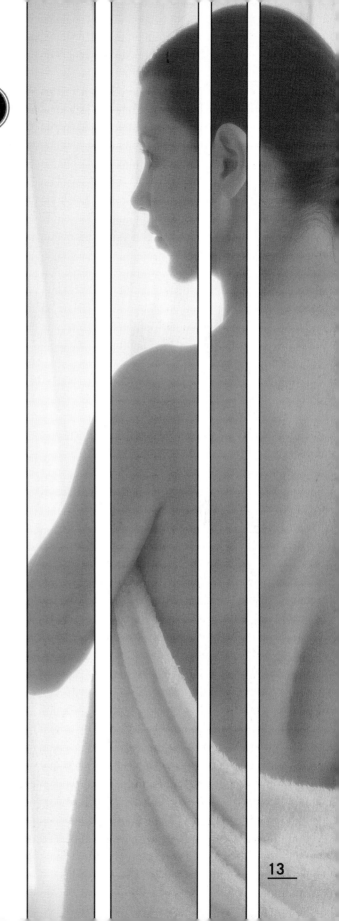

1 Health, safety and hygiene

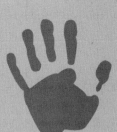

After you have studied this chapter you will be able to:
1. understand the legal requirements under the Health and Safety at Work Act
2. distinguish between hazard and risk
3. explain the role of the Health and Safety Executive (HSE)
4. list the actions that may be taken by the HSE
5. differentiate between health, safety and welfare issues in the workplace
6. discuss the ways of protecting everyone in the workplace from exposure to hazardous substances
7. explain the safety considerations related to electrical equipment
8. understand the importance of reporting injuries, diseases and dangerous occurrences
9. describe the importance of administering first aid in the workplace
10. describe the correct techniques for lifting
11. state the precautions that must be in place to meet fire regulations
12. carry out a risk assessment
13. distinguish between infection and infestation
14. differentiate between bacteria, viruses, fungi and protozoa
15. distinguish between natural immunity and artificial immunity
16. explain the ways in which micro-organisms enter the body and may be transmitted
17. list the required conditions for growth of bacteria
18. distinguish between ectoparasites and endoparasites
19. discuss the factors to be considered in maintaining high standards of salon hygiene
20. discuss the factors to be considered in maintaining high standards of personal hygiene.

Health and safety is about preventing any person sustaining injury, being harmed in any way or becoming ill at work. It involves following correct, safe procedures and taking every possible precaution to protect everyone in the workplace.

Health and safety laws and regulations apply to everyone whether they are employers, managers, employees, self-employed, full- or part-time, paid or unpaid workers. Health and safety issues refer to hazards and risks in the workplace and how to eliminate them.

DEFINITIONS

Hazard means anything that can cause harm.
Risk is the chance, great or small, that someone will be harmed by the hazard.

❖ *Health and Safety at Work Act 1974* ❖

This is the main legislation covering health and safety in the workplace; other safety regulations and codes of practice come under this main Act.

This Act states that employers/managers have a legal duty to ensure, so far as is reasonably practicable, the health, safety and welfare of all persons at work, i.e. all employees and other persons on the premises, such as contractors and clients.

The Health and Safety Executive provides information and publications on all aspects of health and safety regulations, implementing directives from the European Commission that used to be known as the six pack. These cover a wide range of health, safety and welfare issues. Those relevant to the therapist are dealt with in this text.

The Act of 1974 and the new regulations mean that employers must, by law, provide a safe working environment for all members of the workforce, including those with disabilities and other persons using their premises.

Employers are required to:

◎ provide a safe working environment; they must recognise hazards or problems, and take the appropriate actions to minimise or eliminate them

◎ have a written health and safety policy that sets out how these issues are managed

◎ assess the risks that may arise from work activities

◎ record the findings of the risk assessment

◎ consult with colleagues and employees regarding health and safety issues

◎ provide health and safety information, training and supervision for all employees.

The Health and Safety Executive (HSE)

This is a body of people appointed to enforce health and safety law. Inspectors from the Health and Safety Executive or from your Local Authority have the statutory right to inspect your workplace at any time, with or without prior notice. During the visit the inspector will be looking at the premises, the working environment and the work practices. S/he will check that you are complying with health and safety law and will assess whether there are any hazards or risks to the health, safety or welfare of anyone on the premises.

The inspectors can:

◎ inspect all aspects relating to health, safety and welfare

◎ take photographs

◎ ask questions or talk to anyone in the salon

◎ investigate any complaint

◎ offer guidance and advice.

The inspector will ensure that those in charge have arrangements in place for consulting with, training and informing all staff on all matters relating to health, safety and welfare. All staff will be given the opportunity to speak to the inspector privately should they wish to do so. The inspector will provide information and highlight areas of concern to the employers. S/he will also explain why enforcement action is to be taken.

If a breach of the law is found, the inspector will decide what action to take. The action will depend on the severity of the problem.

Actions that may be taken by HSE inspectors

1 *Informal notice*: If the problem is a minor one, the inspector may simply explain what must be done to comply with the law. If asked, s/he will confirm any advice in writing.

2 *Improvement notice*: If the problem is more serious, the inspector may issue an improvement notice. This will state what needs to be done and the time limit by which it must be done. At least 21 days must be allowed for corrective action to be taken.

3 *Prohibition notice*: If the problem poses a serious risk, the inspector may give notice to stop the activity immediately and not allow it to be resumed until corrective action is taken. The notice will explain why such action is necessary.

4 *Prosecution*: A failure to act upon an improvement or prohibition notice may result in prosecution. The courts have the power to impose unlimited fines and, in some severe cases, imprisonment.

An employer has the right of appeal to an industrial tribunal when an improvement or prohibition notice is served should s/he disagree with it or feel that it is unjust. The instructions on how to appeal appear on the back of the notice.

❖ *The therapist's role in maintaining health and safety in their place of work* ❖

The employer/manager is responsible for the management and control of health, safety and welfare issues, which will ensure a safe environment for all persons working in or attending the salon/clinic. However, *all therapists* at work also have a duty under the Act.

Employees are required to:

◎ take reasonable care to avoid harm to themselves or to others by their behaviour or working practices

◎ cooperate with and help employers/managers to meet the statutory requirements

◎ refrain from misusing or interfering with anything provided to protect the health, safety and welfare of all persons as required by the Act.

To comply with these requirements you must:

◎ not put yourself or others at risk by your actions

◎ abide by salon rules and regulations

◎ know who is responsible for what in the salon and to whom you should report problems

◎ always adopt good working practices and follow correct procedures

◎ be alert to any hazard that may pose a risk to yourself or to others and promptly take the appropriate action to minimise or eliminate the risk. If you are unable to, or unsure of how to deal quickly with a hazard, then you must report the situation to someone else immediately. Seek advice from a supervisor or someone qualified to deal with the situation

◎ be competent in selecting appropriate treatments and in administering them correctly and safely to the clients

◎ follow the correct technique for all treatments, understand the effects, and be alert to contra-indications and contra-actions

◎ adopt high professional standards of dress and appearance

◎ maintain the highest standards of personal and salon hygiene

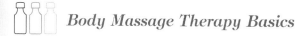

◎ report faulty equipment to the person responsible for dealing with these issues

◎ not ignore any hazard or risk; make sure that corrective action is taken

◎ keep a record of and report any problems that you have identified and rectified

◎ inform your supervisor and colleagues and be prepared to discuss issues of health and safety with all other workers, as shared knowledge makes for a safer working environment.

Health, Safety and Welfare Regulations Applicable to the Massage/Beauty Therapist

The Workplace (Health, Safety and Welfare) Regulations 1992

This regulation covers health, safety and welfare in the workplace.

Workplace means any place where people are employed or are self-employed; it includes the outdoor areas such as paths, etc.

Health issues under this Act include:

ADEQUATE VENTILATION

Premises must be well ventilated, removing stale air and drawing in fresh clean air without draughts.

COMFORTABLE WORKING TEMPERATURE

It is difficult to select the temperature to suit everybody: around 16°C is recommended. The temperature should be comfortable for working but the client will usually be inactive and may feel cold; make sure that s/he is also warm enough.

ADEQUATE LIGHTING

Lighting must be adequate to enable people to work and move around safely. It should be suitable for the treatment in progress; low soft lighting is desirable for some massage routines.

CLEANLINESS AND HYGIENE

Premises must be cleaned regularly to the highest standard. Floors, walls and ceilings together with furniture and fittings should be washed and disinfected where possible. All towels and sheets used should be boil-washed after each client.

Hygiene is discussed later in this chapter.

WASTE

Waste must be stored in suitable, covered bins and disposed of in accordance with regulations. Disposable needles must be placed in a 'sharps box' for collection.

ADEQUATE SPACE FOR WORKING

Cubicles containing a couch, trolley, chair, stools and waste bin should be large enough for the therapist and client to move around in easily. There should be adequate space for all staff to move around easily in the salon without having to negotiate obstacles.

Safety issues under this Act include:

MAINTENANCE OF EQUIPMENT

Everything in the workplace, the equipment and systems, should be maintained in efficient working order. If a fault occurs in any machine or other equipment, it must be taken out of use immediately. It must be clearly labelled 'FAULTY, OUT OF USE' and stored away from the working area. The fault must be reported and the appropriate action taken to repair it.

FLOORS AND TRAFFIC ROUTES

Floors should be sound and even, with a non-slippery surface and must be kept free of obstacles. Any spillages such as water, oil, powder etc, should be wiped up immediately because they will make the floor slippery, which may result in someone slipping and falling. Doors should be wide enough for easy access and exit; stairs should be sound and well lit. A handrail should be provided on at least one side of the stairs.

FALLS AND FALLING OBJECTS

Every effort must be made to prevent anyone falling on the premises. Sound, even, non-slip floors will help. Leads should not trail across the floor but should lie along the wall; stools and bins should be stored under couches; other equipment must not be left around but must be stored correctly.

Every effort must be made to prevent objects falling and injuring people. Storage shelves must be checked regularly and examined for any damage that may weaken them. Objects should be stored and stacked safely in such a way that they are not likely to fall. Shelves should not be overloaded and should have maximum load notices.

WINDOWS

These should be clean and open easily. Ensure that people cannot walk into them if they are open.

Welfare issues under this Act include:

SANITARY CONVENIENCES

Toilets and washing facilities should be available to all persons. These rooms should be clean (cleaned and disinfected regularly), well lit and ventilated. There should be hot and cold running water, soap (preferably in a dispenser), and drying facilities such as paper towels or dry air machines (to prevent the spread of micro-organisms).

DRINKING WATER

An adequate supply of fresh drinking water must be provided, either direct mains water, a chilled water dispenser or bottled water.

CHANGING ROOMS

These rooms must be clean, suitable and secure, where outer garments can be removed and uniforms put on. Changing rooms are also desirable for clients although the cubicles too may be used if privacy for the user can be ensured.

FACILITIES FOR RESTING AND EATING

Food and drink should not be consumed in the treatment cubicles or in the salon. A clean room should be allocated for eating. Adequate comfortable chairs should be provided as well as a table or tables on which to place food and drink.

❖ *Safety considerations when dealing with hazardous substances* ❖

The Control of Substances Hazardous to Health Act 2002 (COSHH)

This law requires employers to control exposure to hazardous substances to prevent ill health. It protects everyone in the workplace from exposure to hazardous substances.

Hazardous substances found in the salon include:

- ◎ cleaning agents
- ◎ disinfectants
- ◎ massage products – oils, creams, lotions and talcum powder
- ◎ powders or dust
- ◎ micro-organisms, i.e. bacteria, viruses, fungi, protozoa
- ◎ parasites
- ◎ ozone.

Hazardous substances can enter the body via many routes, for example:

➤ broken or damaged skin

➤ eyes and ears

➤ nose and mouth

➤ hair follicles.

Substances hazardous to health may cause the following:

◎ skin burn

◎ skin allergic reaction such as dermatitis

◎ skin irritation

◎ irritation of nasal passages and lungs or allergies to products, especially fine powder or dust, resulting in the development of asthma

◎ breathing difficulties

◎ nausea and vomiting if swallowed

◎ eye damage.

COSHH requires you to:

Assess the risk from exposure to hazardous substances to anyone using your workplace. You will need to examine all the substances stored and used in your salon and identify the ones that could cause damage or injury. You will need to consider any risks that these substances present to people's health.

Decide what precautions need to be taken. Check the manufacturers' advice on use, storage and disposal. Read the label carefully. Consider whether the substance can enter the body or damage any part of the body. Take action to protect employees and others. Consider the use of gloves, masks and other protective clothing. Ensure that your control systems are in place and effective.

Control or reduce the exposure to hazardous substances. Consider the use of other, safer, products. Store all products safely and label them clearly to reduce any errors in handling. Wear gloves when handling cleaning agents. Take care when handling and using fine powders such as talc; avoid releasing the fine particles into the air and avoid inhaling any powders; also protect your client.

Ensure that control measures are in place and regularly monitored for effectiveness. Keep records of all control measures and any tests or problems arising. These records should be kept for at least five years.

Prepare procedures to deal with accidents, incidents and emergencies. Immediate steps must be taken to minimise the harmful effects and damage. These procedures should be clearly written and placed in a prominent and accessible place.

Train and supervise all staff. Ensure that all employees understand the risks from all the hazardous substances they have to deal with. Inform them of the rules and regulations for using, storing and transporting or disposing of hazardous substances.

Ensure that all employees understand the importance of reporting any problems or shortcomings when dealing with hazardous substances.

Precautions and responsibilities when dealing with hazardous substances

1 Consider any hazardous substances in your workplace. For the therapist these will include any fine powders such as face powder or talcum powder, oils, creams or lotions, cleaning agents, sterilising agents, micro-organisms, blood.

2 Read the labels and manufacturers' instructions on all the products that you use. Manufacturers are required by law to state the dangers and issue guidelines on storage, use and disposal.

3 Ensure that products are clearly labelled and stored correctly and safely.

4 Ensure that the highest standards of hygiene are implemented to prevent cross-infection (this is dealt with later in the chapter).

5 Avoid blood contamination. Cover any broken skin with a plaster and wear gloves.

6 Ensure the safe disposal of 'sharps' into a 'sharps box' and dispose of in accordance with the correct procedure.

❖ *Safety considerations when using electrical equipment* ❖

The Provision and Use of Work Equipment Regulation 1998

and

The Electricity at Work Regulation 1989

These regulations require that all equipment provided for use at work is:

◎ suitable and safe for the intended use

◎ inspected regularly by a competent person and maintained in a safe condition

◎ used only by therapists who are fully informed, trained and competent in their use.

Therapists use many different types of electrical equipment to treat their clients. It is therefore very important that you understand, and are able to assess, the hazards and risks associated with their use and know what action to take to eliminate or minimise them.

The main hazards and risks are:

H. exposed parts of the leads, wiring or cables
R. contact with these will result in shock or/and burns, which may prove fatal.

H. faulty equipment
R. contact will cause electric shock.

H. faults in the wiring or overloading the circuit
R. may cause fires resulting in injury or even death if the fire is severe.

H. water in the area where electrical equipment is used or working with wet hands
R. electric shock.

H. trailing leads and cables across the floor
R. tripping people up and causing injury.

H. loose-fitting bulbs
R. falling on clients, causing burns or falling on bedding and towels, causing fires.

H. positioning lamps directly over clients
R. falling or exploding bulbs may cause burns and injure the client.

Precautions and responsibilities when using electrical equipment

◎ Annual testing of electrical equipment is required by law.

◎ Ensure that people using electrical equipment are trained and competent to do so.

◎ Follow the correct procedures when using electrical equipment.

◎ Purchase equipment from a reputable dealer who will provide an after-sales service.

◎ Ensure that all equipment is regularly maintained and in a safe condition for use.

◎ Examine leads and cables regularly to ensure that they are without splits or breaks that may expose bare wires.

◎ Use proper connectors to join wire and flexes; do not use insulating tape.

◎ Examine all connections making sure that they are secure.

◎ Ensure that the cable is firmly clamped into the plug to make certain that the wires, particularly the earth wire, cannot be pulled out of the terminal.

◎ Do not overload the circuit by using multiple adaptors. If you find others overloading the circuit, explain to them that this is dangerous practice.

◎ Plug the machine into a near and accessible identified socket so that it can be switched off or disconnected easily in an emergency.

◎ Keep electrical equipment away from water; do not touch any electrical part with wet hands.

◎ Ensure that flexes and cables do not trail over the working area: fix them along the wall.

◎ Examine all equipment regularly, especially portable machines, as they are subjected to wear and tear.

◎ Remove faulty equipment from the working area and label clearly 'FAULTY DO NOT USE' and inform others that it is faulty.

◎ Keep a dated record of when checks were carried out, including all findings and maintenance.

❖ *Reporting of Injuries, Diseases and Dangerous Occurrences Regulations 1985 (RIDDOR)* ❖

This regulation places a legal duty on employers, the self-employed and those in control of premises to report work-related incidents. These incidents must be reported to the Health and Safety Executive (HSE) or your Local Authority (LA).

If you inform the Incident Contact Centre (ICC), they will report and forward the information to the correct enforcing authority on your behalf.

The Incident Contact Centre (ICC)
Caerphilly Business Park
Caerphilly
CF83 3GG
Tel: 0845 300 9923
Website: www.riddor.gov.uk
Email: riddor@natbrit.com
Fax: 0845 300 9924

By law the following incidents must be reported:

◎ deaths

◎ major injuries or poisonings

◎ any accident where the person injured is away from work for more than three days

◎ injuries where members of the public are taken to hospital

◎ diseases contracted at work

◎ dangerous occurrences that did not result in reportable injury but might have done.

❖ *First aid at work* ❖

The Health and Safety (First Aid) Regulations 1981

These regulations require all employers to provide adequate and appropriate equipment, facilities and personnel to enable first aid to be given to employees and others if they are injured or become ill at work.

First aid is the immediate treatment administered when any person suffers an injury or becomes ill at work. The minimum first aid provision at any workplace includes:

◎ a suitably stocked first aid box placed in a precise, easily accessible and clearly labelled site

◎ an appointed person to take charge of first aid arrangements.

First aid provision must be available at all times to people at work. It may therefore be necessary to train more than one person to be in charge.

The duties of the appointed first aid person will include:

◎ taking charge and administering appropriate treatment (providing that they have been trained to do so) when someone is injured or falls ill

◎ calling an ambulance if required, depending on the seriousness of the injury

◎ taking responsibility for the contents of the first aid box and restocking as required.

The designated first aid person must have received training in administering first aid and hold a current first aid certificate.

Appointed persons should not give first aid for which they have not been trained. Short emergency first aid training courses are available. This training must have the approval of the HSE.

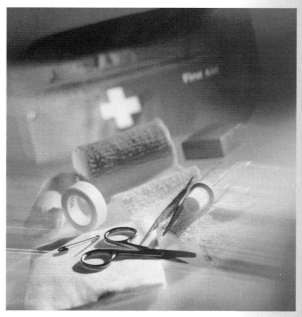

Figure 1.1   First aid box.

All *employees* must be informed of the first aid arrangements. Notices situated in clearly visible places must inform them of who and where the appointed first aid persons are, and where the first aid box is located.

Remember to check the contents of the first aid box regularly. Write a list of the items in the box when it is new and use as your check list.

❖ *Manual handling* ❖

The Manual Handling Operations Regulations 1992

This regulation requires all employers to assess the risk to employees when lifting or handling heavy goods and to provide training in safe techniques.

More than a third of all over-three-day injuries reported each year to the HSE and LAs are caused by manual handling, i.e. lifting, transporting or supporting loads by hand or bodily force. The accidents primarily result in back injuries, but hands, arms and feet may also be injured. These injuries may build up over time as a result of repetitive movements or may be caused by single poor-lifting techniques or too heavy a load. As a therapist you may be required to receive, check and handle deliveries and transport these to the stock room, or to move couches in the salon. It is therefore essential that you are able to assess the risk and protect yourself from injury.

Before lifting or moving anything:

Assess the risk:

- how heavy is the load
- can you reduce the load
- do you have to lift it off the floor – this produces the greatest risk
- can you get assistance from another person
- how far do you have to move it
- can you rest it halfway on a chair or table to ease the effort?

LIFTING TECHNIQUES

- Feet apart on either side of the load for a balanced stable base
- Good posture; maintain natural curves
- Tuck chin in, keep a straight back, lower and bend the knees
- Take a firm grip

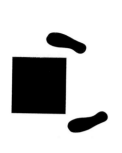 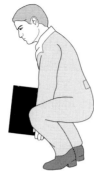

Figure 1.2 Feet on either side of the load for a stable base.

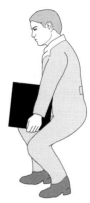

Figure 1.3 Bend the knees and keep the arms into the sides.

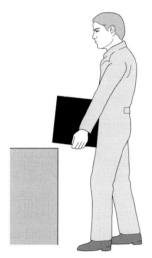

Figure 1.4 Take a firm grip and hold the load close to the body.

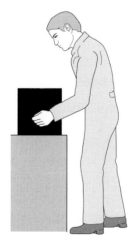

Figure 1.5 Lift smoothly. Do not twist the trunk when placing the load down.

➤ Keep the arms into the sides; hold the load close to the body. If you hold it away from the body, this increases the leverage and risk of injury

➤ Lift smoothly; do not jerk or twist the body as you lift. Move the feet and place the load in position

➤ Do not twist the trunk when placing the load down

➤ Back strains and injuries can also occur as a result of incorrect posture and stance when performing massage. Ensure that you adopt the correct stance. Keep the back straight and bend the knees; do not twist the body as you work and avoid stretching over the client.

Remember, do not put yourself or others at risk.

❖ *Fire precautions* ❖

The Fire Precautions (Workplace) Regulations 1997

These regulations require the employer to ensure that safety measures are in place to prevent and deal with the outbreak of fire in the salon. S/he must assess the fire risks, keep a written record of these risks and inform all employees of the findings. The following precautions and measures must be in place:

- ◎ Smoke alarms or other fire detection equipment must be fitted, checked regularly and maintained in good working order.

- ◎ Fire fighting equipment must be in good working order and suitable for the type of fire.

- ◎ Fire fighting equipment must be clearly visible and easily accessible.

- ◎ Fire doors should be fitted if the risk of fire is assessed as high.

- ◎ A means of escape must be provided and marked 'fire exit'.

- ◎ Doors should be left unlocked and kept free of obstruction for quick escape.

- ◎ All employees must be kept informed and trained in fire procedures.

- ◎ Notices for fire procedures and evacuation should be clear and prominently displayed.

Fire is a hazard in any place of work and it is very important that you familiarise yourself with your salon's fire procedures and evacuation drill. If a fire occurs you will need to act very quickly; it is therefore very important to know exactly what to do to ensure your own safety and the safety of others. Remember, others may panic and so it is important that you stay calm and take control of the situation. Knowing exactly what procedure to take beforehand will enable you to act promptly.

All members of staff should ensure that they receive training in fire drill and fire evacuation procedures.

Fire evacuation procedures must be practised regularly.

All staff should know:

- ◎ how to recognise the fire or smoke alarm

- ◎ who to report to and how to raise the alarm

- ◎ how to contact the emergency services or inform the person who is responsible for doing this

- ◎ the exact position of the fire fighting equipment and how to use it should the fire be small and easy to control

- ◎ the colour coding on the fire extinguishers in your salon and what type of fire they are suitable for (these are not included in this text as they may change in the future but ensure that you check all those in your salon). Read the instructions on each one and, if you are unsure of any detail, ask the supervisor or the person responsible

◎ where the exit doors and exit routes are and in what order the salon is to be evacuated

◎ what and how checks are to be made on the numbers of staff and clients or others to ensure that everyone is safe

◎ how you may contain the fire and limit the damage by closing any doors other than exit doors, closing windows, switching off electrical equipment and using a fire blanket to smother the fire. These actions must only be taken if it is safe to do so and would not put yourself or anyone else at risk.

Identify anything that may be a fire hazard in your workplace and take every precaution to avoid risk to yourself and others.

Draw a plan of the position of all the fire fighting equipment in your workplace. Label each piece, state its colour coding and the type of fire it is suitable for.

❖ *Risk assessment* ❖

You may be required to carry out a risk assessment in your workplace to ensure that everything possible is in place to prevent anyone being harmed or contracting illness. It is a legal requirement to keep a written record of the risk assessment if there are five or more employees but it is good practice to do so anyway. You must be able to identify hazards, risks and aspects in your workplace that could cause harm to yourself or others. Consider the following: safe maintenance, care and use of equipment; the safe use, handling and storage of hazardous substances; safe and hygienic working practices; personal and salon hygiene; adequate procedures for dealing with emergencies such as fire, shock etc; proper environmental and welfare requirements.

Procedure

Walk around your salon looking for all the hazards that pose a risk of harm to anyone entering the salon. Consider the hazards mentioned in this text, or any others. Ask colleagues if they have identified anything that may pose a risk. List all the hazards that you have identified.

Check the procedures and controls already in place and ensure that they meet legal requirements.

List the hazards and risks that require action and state the action needed to eliminate them. Give priority to high risks, those that may cause the most serious damage and those that affect the greatest number of people. These should receive immediate attention. Inform all staff of your findings and ensure that they are trained in the new procedures. Set a date for the next risk assessment. Keep a record of the risk assessment in an easily accessible identified place.

Table 1.1   Example record card for risk assessment

Name of workplace:		Signed: .... Date:	
List the significant hazards	List the groups of people who are at risk	List the existing controls or note where they can be found	List and date the actions to be taken to introduce effective controls

The Local Government (Miscellaneous Provisions) Act 1982

Local Authorities issue licences and register businesses offering beauty therapy treatments including massage. They also issue regulations with which, by law, you must comply. Before setting up a business you must contact your Local Authority to ensure that you comply with the exact requirements. When you meet all the requirements you will be issued with a *certificate of registration*. These bye-laws are mainly concerned with issues of hygiene and safety as explained in this text. Environmental health officers have the right under this law to inspect your business and can issue fines or withdraw your registration if you are not complying with the regulations.

Contact your Local Authority and ask for the regulations relating to setting up a business offering massage.

❖ *Hygiene* ❖

Hygiene deals with the precautions and procedures necessary for maintaining health and preventing the spread of disease. In the salon the highest priority must be given to preventing infection, cross-infection and infestation. The massage therapist carries a heavy responsibility for protecting him/herself, other staff and the clients from the risk of contamination by micro-organisms that cause disease.

Infection

An infection or infectious disease is caused by micro-organisms invading the body. The symptoms and severity of the illness will depend on the type of invading micro-organism and the part of the body affected.

Infestation

An infestation is the invasion of the body by animal parasites such as lice, worms, flukes etc; they may live in or on the body. Some parasites merely cause itchy irritation while others cause serious illness.

Micro-organisms or microbes

There are many different types of micro-organism present in the environment. The main groups include:

◎ bacteria

◎ viruses

◎ fungi, yeasts

◎ protozoa.

Micro-organisms entering the body do not always produce disease, as the immune system is stimulated to protect the body. However, if the invading organisms are in large enough numbers to overcome the immune system then disease and illness will occur. Disease will also occur if the body has little immunity to the invading microbes or if the immune system has itself been damaged by disease as in AIDS. If the body's defences are overcome then the microbes will cause damage to or destruction of the cells. Some microbes release toxins that destroy the cells, while others multiply and directly destroy them. The various micro-organisms produce a wide variety of diseases, each one showing particular symptoms. When the immune system fails to contain a disease, drugs are necessary to treat the infections. Antibacterial or antibiotic drugs are used to treat bacterial infections; antiviral drugs to treat viral infections; antifungal drugs to treat fungal and yeast infections; and antiprotozoal drugs to treat infections by protozoa.

Immunity

Natural active immunity

This is obtained when a person comes into contact with a particular microbe and produces antibodies to repel and control it. The antibodies produced to fight that infection remain in the body to control any future infection. Many infectious diseases occur only once in a lifetime, as immunity is lifelong, while others may recur, as immunity may last for only a few years.

Natural passive immunity

This involves the transfer of antibodies from an immunised donor to a recipient. Immunity may be passed from mother to baby via placenta or mother's milk.

Artificial active immunity

Artificial immunity can be provided by the use of vaccines. These are prepared from altered or diluted forms of the organism. Once they are introduced into the body they stimulate the immune system in the same way as an infection but are not strong enough to cause the disease.

Artificial passive immunity

Another type of immunisation that relies on transferring antibodies from someone who has recovered from that particular disease. The transfer is made via a serum containing the antibodies.

Invasion of the body

Micro-organisms enter the body via many routes:

a) through broken or damaged skin

b) through orifices such as the nose, mouth, anus, vagina, urethra

c) through eyes and ears

d) into hair follicles

e) into the bloodstream by blood-sucking insects such as mosquitoes and lice.

Some micro-organisms produce immediate symptoms while others can lie dormant for a long time and attack when the body's immune system is low.

Transmission

Micro-organisms can be transmitted in many ways:

a) By droplet infection: an infected person coughing and sneezing or spitting will expel organisms into the air where they may be inhaled by others.

b) By handling contaminated articles such as clothing, towels and equipment, when micro-organisms may be transmitted to the handler.

c) Dirty surfaces or dusty atmospheres will contain micro-organisms, which may be inhaled or may enter via the eyes or ears.

d) Organisms present in faeces and urine may be transferred to others if the hands are not thoroughly washed after use of the toilet.

e) Food may become contaminated by handling with unwashed hands and flies carrying contamination from excreta and rubbish. Water may become contaminated and then organisms will be transmitted through eating and drinking these foods.

f) Organisms may be spread through contact with animals.

g) Through direct contact with others, hand contact or touching.

h) Organisms may be spread through an intermediary host such as fleas and blood-sucking insects.

i) Contaminated blood, if transmitted to another person, can cause serious and sometimes fatal illness. Organisms can be transmitted through blood transfusion, infected needles or at any time when the blood of the carrier (infected person) enters the body of the recipient. Hepatitis B and the HIV virus, which causes AIDS, are transmitted in this way. These are very serious life-threatening illnesses and great care must be taken to avoid any blood contact at any time. Any blood spots should be dealt with by wearing gloves and using strong disinfectant, e.g. household bleach. Needles and ear piercing equipment must be carefully disposed of into a 'sharps box'.

The conditions required for the growth of micro-organisms are:

1 a food supply

2 a water supply or moisture

3 warmth: pathogenic bacteria favour a body temperature of 37°C. Low temperatures found in the refrigerator or freezer will prevent growth of bacteria but will not destroy them

4 dark conditions: strong UVL will kill bacteria

5 oxygen is required by some bacteria for aerobic respiration but others are anaerobic and survive without oxygen

6 slightly alkaline conditions. (The acidity of the skin – acid mantle – helps to protect against growth of bacteria.)

Ways in which the body resists infection

a) Unbroken skin forms a physical barrier.

b) Mucous membranes, mucus, hairs and cilia help to trap and filter microbes.

c) Saliva washes microbes from teeth and mouths.

d) Tears wash microbes from the eyes.

e) Urine washes microbes from the urethra.

f) Faeces remove microbes from the bowel.

g) The acidic pH of the skin limits growth of bacteria.

h) Sebum produces an oily film that protects the skin.

i) Gastric juices destroy bacteria in the stomach.

j) Various antibodies are produced by the body in response to infection.

k) Macrophages and granulocytes ingest and destroy micro-organisms by a process of phagocytosis.

The *main groups of micro-organisms* that may be found in your workplace are:

Bacteria

Bacteria are single-cell organisms varying in size from $0.2\,\mu m$ to $2.0\,\mu m$ in diameter. They are found everywhere in the environment but can only be seen through an optical microscope. Many bacteria are harmless and useful to humans and are called *non-pathogenic bacteria*. Some are used in the production of food such as cheese and yoghurt. Others help to dispose of unwanted organic material such as the breakdown of sewage, rendering it harmless. Some bacteria in the human intestine help to synthesise vitamins K and B_2. The harmful bacteria that cause disease are known as *pathogenic* or *pathogens*. Bacteria are the simplest of

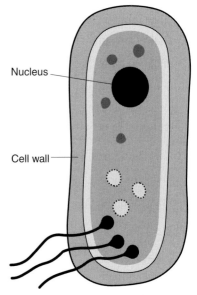

Nucleus

Cell wall

Figure 1.6   A bacterium.

living organisms, composed of a single cell with cytoplasm surrounded by a protective cell membrane but devoid of organelles. They multiply rapidly by dividing into two, known as **binary fission**. This can occur every 20 minutes and a single bacterium may give rise to 16 million bacteria per day. Some bacteria have whip-like projections on the surface of the cell, called flagella: these enable the bacteria to move around. Bacteria may be aerobic, requiring oxygen to sustain life, or they may be anaerobic, able to survive without oxygen.

The aerobic variety is found invading surface tissues of the skin and mucous membranes of the respiratory tract. The anaerobic variety is found in the bowel or deep wounds. Some bacteria develop into spores; these can lie dormant for long periods of time and become active when conditions are suitable. Spores develop a hard, thick outer shell that protects the contents and makes them very difficult to destroy. They are more resistant to heat and disinfectants; higher temperatures and strong chemical disinfectants are required to kill spores.

Bacteria cause disease by producing toxins or poisons that are harmful to body cells. They grow and multiply if the conditions are right.

Types of bacterium

Bacteria are classified according to their shape:

1   *Cocci*: these spherical-shaped bacteria may form clusters known as staphylococci, or chains known as streptococci, or pairs known as diplococci. They can cause a wide variety of conditions such as boils, carbuncles, impetigo, sore throat, meningitis, pneumonia etc.

2   *Bacilli*: these rod-shaped bacteria cause serious illness such as diphtheria, tuberculosis, and typhoid fever.

3   *Spirochetes*: these spiral- or curved-shaped bacteria include spirillium and vibros and cause venereal disease such as syphilis, and serious disease such as cholera.

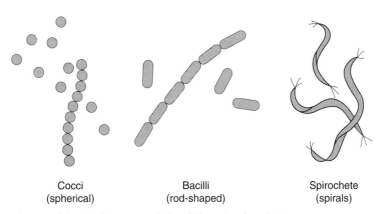

Cocci
(spherical)

Bacilli
(rod-shaped)

Spirochete
(spirals)

Figure 1.7   Three types of bacterium: cocci, bacilli and spirochete.

The body protects itself against bacterial infection by several methods:

a) By producing antitoxins that neutralise toxins produced by the bacteria.

b) By producing large numbers of white cells, macrophages and granulocytes, which circulate in the blood and which engulf and destroy bacteria.

c) By producing antibodies that attack and destroy the bacteria.

The discovery of penicillin and development of other antibiotics and antibacterials mean that bacterial infections can usually be brought under control. Antibiotics must be used in adequate doses for at least five days. Some antibiotics kill the bacteria directly while others prevent multiplication of the bacteria.

Viruses

Viruses are the smallest known infective particles: smaller than bacteria, they can only be seen through an electron microscope. They are between 0.1 μm and 0.2 μm in size, and vary in shape from spheres, cubes or rods.

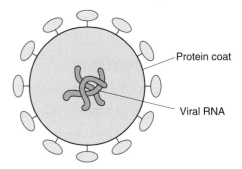

Figure 1.8　A virus.

They consist of a core of nucleic acid, RNA or DNA, enclosed in a protein shell or capsid. Viruses cannot metabolise nor reproduce: they are parasitic, living inside a host cell. Once inside a host cell, a virus causes the host cell to make copies of the virus. Eventually, the host cell is destroyed and hundreds of new viruses released that attack other cells. After the virus enters the host cell there is a period of incubation when the host cells show no sign of disease. Many cycles of viral spread occur and more and more host cells are affected; eventually typical signs and symptoms of the disease occur. By the time the symptoms appear, the viruses are so numerous that antiviral drugs have limited effect. The body protects itself against viral infection by producing specific antibodies. These will also provide future immunity to some diseases; immunity can be produced artificially to combat some viral infections.

Body cells also produce 'interferons', which interfere with the multiplication of viruses. Antiviral drugs are now available, some of which prevent the multiplication of viruses while others alter the DNA within the cell, preventing the virus from using it. In this way the spread of infection is halted.

Viral diseases include the common cold, influenza, poliomyelitis, mumps, herpes simplex and zoster, chicken pox, warts, hepatitis and AIDS.

The Hepatitis B virus and the Human Immunodeficiency Virus (HIV), which causes AIDS, are the two most serious viral infections that could be transmitted between clients and staff in the salon. Both are carried in the blood: even minute amounts of blood or organic material, which may not be visible to the naked eye, can carry the viruses. People may be unaware that they are infected: there are thousands of symptomless carriers worldwide. The particular danger to the therapist and her/his clients is contact with blood or tissue fluid through cuts or abrasions in the skin or anything that pierces the skin.

The correct hygiene procedures must be adhered to to prevent any possibility of infection (see page 40).

Fungi

Fungi are larger than bacteria: they may be unicellular as in yeasts or multicellular as in moulds. The cells contain nuclei and other cell components but do not contain chlorophyll. They obtain their food by secreting enzymes through the cell walls: this digests any organic matter, which is then absorbed as liquid food. Fungi may be *saprophytes*, which obtain food from dead organic matter or they may be *parasites*, which live off plants, animals or humans, feeding off skin and mucous membranes and producing diseases. They reproduce by forming spores. The unicellular fungi and spores are not visible to the naked eye but the filamentous fungi forming mycelia are visible, e.g. moulds and mildews.

Diseases caused by fungi:

1 *Ringworm*: this may affect different parts of the body and is named according to the part affected.
Ringworm of the *foot* is *tinea pedis* (athlete's foot)
Ringworm of the *body* is *tinea corporis*

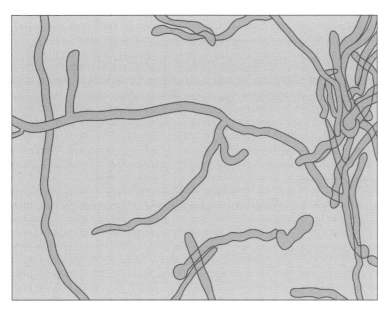

Figure 1.9 Fungi.

Ringworm of the *head* is *tinea capitis*

Ringworm of the *nail* is *tinea unguium*.

2   *Thrush*, which is caused by the fungus Candida albicans.

3   More serious internal fungal infections of the lungs and heart can be fatal.

Once fungal infections invade the body and grow, anti-fungal drugs are required to control the infection as the condition will rarely improve without drugs. Some anti-fungal drugs are applied on to the areas while others are taken by mouth. They destroy the fungal cell wall and the cell dies.

Protozoa

These are the simplest of single-celled animals, slightly bigger than bacteria. Each protozoa is composed of cytoplasm containing a nucleus and organelles surrounded by a cell wall or membrane.They move around by pushing out pseudopodia. Many types are known to exist as parasites on humans, particularly in the bowel. Some are harmless, causing few symptoms; others cause different types of illness, some very serious depending on the organism involved.

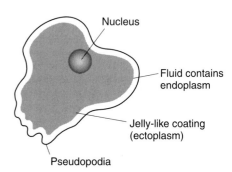

Figure 1.10   Protozoa.

Protozoa may be transmitted from contaminated food and water, through sexual contact and by bites from insects.

Protozoa may infect the bowel causing diarrhoea, general ill health and malaise or they may cause serious illness such as sleeping sickness, malaria, or amoebic dysentery. Treatment requires anti-protozoal drugs to be given over a long period of time as protozoa are difficult to eradicate.

Animal parasites

Parasites are living organisms that live in or on another living organism and derive their food supply from that host.

Ectoparasites live outside the host, e.g. lice, fleas.

Endoparasites live inside the host, e.g. tapeworms or threadworms, roundworms and flukes.

The presence of any parasite on the body is known as an **infestation**.

Ectoparasites

1 Head lice (Pediculus capitis)

The head louse is an insect found on the human scalp. It obtains its nourishment by piercing the skin and sucking blood. The adult female is slightly larger than the male, about 2 mm–3 mm long and 1 mm wide. The female lays white, shiny oval-shaped eggs called nits; they are cemented to the hair close to the scalp. They take approximately 1 week to mature and can reproduce in another week. The life cycle of a louse lasts for 4–5 weeks during which time the female will lay around 300 eggs. They cause intense itching, and secondary infections may result due to scratching. Lice and nits may be killed by special shampoos or lotions containing insecticide and combing out with a fine tooth comb.

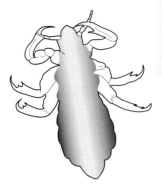

Figure 1.11   Head louse.

2 Body lice (Pediculus corporis)

These are similar to but larger than head lice. They obtain nutrients by sucking blood and laying eggs in underclothing. The crab louse is smaller and is found in pubic and underarm hair. Treatment is by insecticidal shampoo, and clothing, towels, etc. that have been in contact must be washed in insecticidal soap and boil-washed.

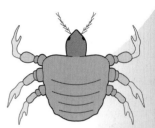

Figure 1.12   Body louse.

3 Itch mites (Sarcoptes scabies)

This is a tiny animal that burrows into the skin producing a condition called scabies. It has 8 legs and is around 0.3 mm long and 0.2 mm wide. The fertilised female burrows into the skin forming dark lines about 1 cm long. She lays around 60 eggs in the burrows, which hatch in 4–8 days. The burrows are seen between the fingers, on the front of the wrists, forearms or may be on male genitalia. They cause intense irritation, vesicles, papules and pustules. They are easily passed from person to person. Medical opinion should be sought and any clothing, towels etc that have come into contact with such a client must be burned.

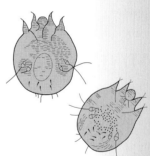

Figure 1.13   Itch mite.

4 Fleas

The flea is an insect with 3 pairs of legs that enable it to jump long distances from host to host. It obtains nourishment by biting and sucking the blood of the host. The bites cause red spots usually found in groups; they are intensely itchy.

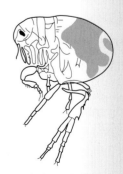

Figure 1.14   A flea.

Fleas lay eggs in dust, carpets or furniture. They can be eliminated by spraying with insecticides, washing clothing and bedding and thorough cleaning of soft furnishings. The flea was responsible for carrying the plague.

Endoparasites

These include a variety of worms and flukes. Infestation is usually the result of poor standards of hygiene and insanitary conditions. Worms may be passed on to humans through contaminated food or water, while undercooked pork and beef are a source of tapeworms. Threadworms, tapeworms and roundworms live in the intestine and may cause diarrhoea, weakness and anaemia. Liver flukes live in the bile ducts and liver, causing jaundice, while

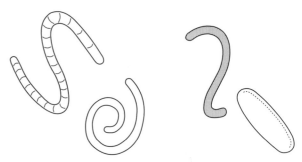

Figure 1.15   Worms and flukes.

some serious types of fluke invade small blood vessels, causing serious illness.

The body's defences are not effective against these infestations and drug treatment is essential to eliminate the worms.

These anthelmintic drugs kill or paralyse the worms and they pass out of the body in faeces. If serious complications have occurred, other drugs may be necessary to deal with these.

Methods of controlling micro-organisms

The process of controlling micro-organisms in the salon is the responsibility of all therapists and must be taken seriously. Correct hygiene procedures must be adopted as a matter of routine. Any instruments and equipment used must always be cleaned after use then sterilised or disinfected.

Various words are used to explain hygiene procedures. Their meaning must be clearly understood so that the appropriate methods are selected. British Standard definitions are as follows:

Antibiotic. An organic chemical substance that, in dilute solution, can destroy or inhibit growth of bacteria and some other micro-organisms. Antibiotics are used to treat infectious diseases in humans, animals and plants.

Antiseptic. A chemical agent that destroys or inhibits growth of micro-organisms on living tissues, thus limiting or preventing the harmful results of infection (usually used on wounds, sores or skin cleansing).

Aseptic methods. Procedures adopted for creating conditions for avoiding infection.

Bactericide. A chemical agent that, under defined conditions, is capable of killing bacteria but not necessarily the spores.

Bacteriostat/fungistat. Chemical agents that, under defined conditions, are capable of inhibiting the multiplication of bacteria/fungi.

Biocide, fungicide, virucide, sporicide. These words imply the destruction of bacteria, fungi, viruses and spores. Biocide kills everything.

Disinfectant. A chemical agent that destroys micro-organisms but not spores (usually used on articles, implements, surfaces, drains etc).

Sanitation. The establishment of conditions favourable to health and preventing the spread of disease.

Sepsis/septic. Being infected by bacteria usually associated with pus formation.

Sterilisation. The total destruction or removal of all living micro-organisms and their spores.

Procedures to prevent cross-infection in the salon

While it is impossible to create a perfectly sterile environment in the salon, every effort must be made to limit the growth and to destroy micro-organisms by practising high standards of hygiene. *Procedures must be in place and adhered to, in order to protect yourself, other therapists and clients from cross-infection.* This is a legal requirement.

1 Hands *must* be washed frequently, before touching every client and after treatment, after handling equipment and after using the toilet. A bactericidal product such as Hibiscrub should be used. Hands should be dried with a disposable towel or hot air dryer.

2 Nails must be kept short and clean to prevent harbouring micro-organisms under the nail.

3 Hands and nails must be examined for any cuts and abrasions or infections. If small, they may be covered with a waterproof plaster and fingerstall.

4 Therapists or clients with any infection or infestation should not give or receive treatment until the conditions have been medically treated and cured.

5 All clients should shower and the client's skin should be cleaned before treatment with surgical spirit or Savlon wipes. Any cuts and abrasions must be covered with a waterproof plaster.

6 Clean towels and sheets must be provided for every client; these should be carefully removed after treatment and placed in a laundry basket/bin. They should be *boil-washed after each client*. Therefore a plentiful supply of good-quality towels should be available for covering the couch and for client use. Disposable paper sheets should be used to protect the towelling couch cover and disposed of after each client.

7   Commodities should be chosen with care; creams, lotions, oils etc should preferably be contained in dispensers, or failing this, in tubes or narrow-necked bottles, which have a smaller surface to be contaminated than wide-necked jars.

8   A new clean spatula must be used to remove creams or lotions from jars; do not return any contaminated article back to the product. Lift the required amount of product in one scoop if possible and place it on a dish ready for use. Wash and disinfect the dish after use.

9   If bleeding occurs for any reason, even the smallest amount must be dealt with immediately. Do not touch the blood; wear rubber gloves. Clean the skin with a sterile dressing and cover with a waterproof dressing. If there is blood on any surface such as the couch or floor, pour on neat chlorine, e.g. Domestos, leave for 10 minutes then wipe off with a disposable cloth. Wash with water and detergent and wipe over with more Domestos. Dispose of the cloth and gloves into a plastic bin bag.

10 The salon should always be clean, neat and tidy. All surfaces should be wiped down frequently during the day using 70% alcohol or products such as Dispray. At the end of each day they should be washed down with water and detergent and wiped over with 10% Domestos. Chairs, stools, couches, trolleys should also be cleaned in this way at the end of the day.

11 Bins with plastic liners should be easily reached. All waste should be immediately disposed of; wet waste should first be wrapped in paper. The waste bins should be emptied and disinfected every night and clean liners inserted.

12 Any articles used must be thoroughly clean before being sterilised or disinfected. The articles should be thoroughly soaked, washed and scrubbed with a hard brush in water and detergent. Care must be taken to reach the more inaccessible parts so that all matter is removed. Finally, they should be rinsed thoroughly under running water then disinfected or sterilised as appropriate.
    (Although the massage therapist will not be required to use such equipment they should be aware that a special sharps box should be available for disposal of needles, razors etc. that could penetrate the skin. Special arrangement for collection and subsequent disposal of these boxes can be organised by contacting the local environmental health officer.)

13 Toilet and hand washing facilities should be easily accessible. These should be well ventilated and disinfected at least once a day. Sanitary ware and floors can be cleaned using Domestos in the correct dilution.

14 A cloakroom should be available for leaving outdoor clothes and changing into uniform. This reduces the risk of carrying micro-organisms from the outside into the salon.

Cleaning of equipment

Sterilisation will destroy micro-organisms and spores

Sterilisation is the best procedure for small articles and instruments and should be a major consideration when purchasing these articles. The therapist should check with the manufacturer that the materials are suitable for the chosen method of sterilisation. Instruments made of stainless steel and certain plastics are suitable, although sharp edges may be blunted by exposure to heat.

Methods of sterilising used in salons include:

- ultraviolet light cabinets
- glass bead steriliser
- dry-heat ovens
- autoclave/moist heat
- sterilising liquids.

Disinfectants

Disinfection will destroy micro-organisms but not spores

Equipment made from materials that are not suitable for sterilisation must be disinfected. Also shelves, work surfaces and other surfaces should be regularly wiped over with disinfectant solutions.

A wide variety of products is available and any information regarding the products should be carefully studied in order to make an informed choice. Follow the manufacturer's instructions, use with care and protect your skin with gloves. Disinfectants must be used in the concentrations recommended; if they are further diluted their effectiveness is reduced. Most disinfectants are more effective at higher temperatures.

Other factors that may reduce effectiveness are:

1   the presence of organic matter such as dead skin, dried blood or vomit; as previously stated, all articles should be cleaned before disinfection

2   some disinfectants are inactivated by hard water while others are inactivated by soaps

3   effectiveness is progressively diminished with age. Store only for the recommended time; do not use after the expiry date.

Disinfectants, if incorrectly stored, used and diluted can themselves become infected and be a source of infection.

Suggested uses:

- → for soaking and immersion of implements – Cydex and Milton
- → wiping VS cups and electrodes – surgical spirit, Isopropyl, salon wipes, alcohol
- → cleaning surfaces – Dettinox, Dispray, Domestos
- → cleaning skin – surgical spirit, Savlon
- → washing hands – Hibiscrub and other bactericidal soaps
- → toilets and sanitary ware – Dettol, Izal, Domestos.

Summary

If micro-organisms invade the body in sufficient numbers to overcome the immune system they will cause disease.

Micro-organisms that infect the body are bacteria, viruses, fungi or yeasts and protozoa.

Immunity

1 *Natural immunity*: acquired by previous contact with disease: antibodies remain in the body or are acquired via the placenta or milk from the mother.

2 *Artificial immunity*: acquired from vaccines introduced into the body that stimulate the immune system to produce antibodies or may be acquired by transfer of antibodies from a person who has recovered from the disease.

Bacteria: single-cell organisms, non-pathogenic – cocci, bacilli, spirochetes.

Diseases caused by bacteria: boils, impetigo, sore throat, meningitis, pneumonia, typhoid fever, syphilis, cholera.

Viruses: invade, multiply and destroy the host cells.

Diseases caused by viruses: colds, influenza, glandular fever, poliomyelitis, mumps, measles, chicken pox, herpes simplex and herpes zoster, warts, verruca, hepatitis, AIDS. The hepatitis B virus and HIV (AIDS) virus found in semen, saliva and blood may be transmitted through blood transfusion, drug users sharing needles, or transfer of blood or body fluids from an infected person into a recipient via a cut or puncture of the skin; infected women may pass it to the foetus.

Fungi: yeasts and moulds.

Diseases caused by fungi: tinea of various parts of the body, thrush, fungal infections of organs such as heart and lungs.

Health, safety and hygiene

Protozoa: single-celled animals.

Diseases caused by protozoa: sleeping sickness, malaria, amoebic dysentery.

Parasites live in or on another living organism:

1　Ectoparasites live outside host, e.g. lice and fleas.

2　Endoparasites live inside host, e.g. worms and flukes.

Sterilisation is the total destruction of microbes and spores.

Disinfecting: use of a chemical agent that destroys microbes but not spores.

Disinfectants for use in salon:
- 70% alcohol

    – methylated spirit and surgical spirit

    – isopropyl alcohol

- glutaraldehyde – Cydex
- chlorine – Milton, Domestos
- phenols – Dettol, Dettinox, Izal, Lysol
- ammonium compounds – Cetavlon, Savlon
- diquamides – Hibitane, Hibiscrub, Dispray

Q U E S T I O N S

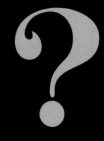

1. Define (a) hazard and (b) risk.
2. What is the role of the Health and Safety Executive (HSE)?
3. List the actions that can be taken by the inspector if a breach in the law is found during an inspection.
4. Explain the actions you would take if you discovered a hazard in the workplace that might pose a risk to yourself or others.
5. Explain the *health* precautions you would consider in the salon in order to comply with the health, safety and welfare regulations.
6. Explain the *safety* precautions you would

consider in order to comply with the health, safety and welfare regulations.

7. Explain the *welfare* precautions you would consider in order to comply with the health, safety and welfare regulations.

8. What does COSHH stand for?

9. List five hazardous substances that may be found in the salon.

10. Give three legal requirements relating to the safe use of electrical equipment.

11. List any five hazards that may be found in the salon and explain their associated risks.

12. List ten precautions and responsibilities when using electrical equipment.

13. State the employer's responsibility under the First Aid Regulations 1981.

14. State the minimum first aid provision under the Act.

15. Define the terms 'infection' and 'infestation'.

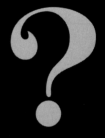

16. Explain briefly how bacteria and viruses multiply.

17. Name three diseases caused by each of the following:
    (a) bacteria
    (b) viruses
    (c) fungi
    (d) protozoa.

18. Explain the term 'natural active immunity'.

19. Give two methods of producing artificial immunity.

20. List five ways in which microbes may enter the body.

21. Explain how microbes may be transmitted.

22. Explain how Hepatitis B and HIV (AIDS) may be transmitted.

23. Define the terms 'ectoparasite' and 'endoparasite' and give three examples of each.

24. Define the following:
    (a) sterilisation
    (b) sanitation
    (c) disinfectant
    (d) antiseptic
    (e) bactericide
    (f) biocide.

Note: Guideline answers to the questions in this chapter only are to be found on pages 306–308.

2 Body systems and the physiological and psychological effects of massage

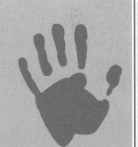

O B J E C T I V E S

After you have studied this chapter you will be able to:
1. describe the organisational levels of the body
2. list the classification of tissues
3. list the types of epithelial tissue and state where they are found
4. list the types of connective tissue and give their function
5. list the body systems and
   a) describe the main body systems relevant to massage
   b) explain the functions of these systems
   c) explain the physiological effects of massage on the main body systems
   d) explain the psychological effects of massage.

❖ *Organisational levels* ❖

Massage is applied directly to the body and produces effects on the body tissues. An understanding of the structure of the body and how it functions is therefore essential to plan effective treatments and explain them to the client.

Anatomy is the study of the structure of the body.

Physiology is the study of how the body functions.

The following section will provide you with basic information relating to the structure and function of each of the body systems and will explain the effects of massage on each one. The body is made up of billions of cells containing chemical elements that carry out all the functions that are essential for maintaining life. These cells group together to form tissues,

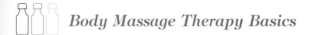

which further group together to form the body organs; many organs join together to form the systems of the body. We can study these organisational levels in greater detail.

The organisational levels are:

chemical—cell—tissue—organ—system

Chemical

At the very basic level are the **chemical** substances within the cell. Reactions in which these chemicals combine or break down underlie all the processes essential for life.

Cells

These are the basic structural and functional units of the body. All the activities that maintain life are carried out by the **cells**. The body is made up of billions of cells; they all have a similar structure, but are modified to suit their function, e.g. blood cells differ from fat cells.

Tissues

Groups of similar cells form the **tissues** of the body. All the cells of one tissue will be identical, but will be different for different tissues, e.g. epithelial tissue covers the body and skeletal muscle tissue produces movement.

Organs

Different tissues group together to form the **organs** of the body. Each organ will perform a specific function, e.g. the heart pumps blood around the body.

Systems

Many different organs link together to form the **systems** of the body. They work together to carry out an essential function, e.g. the digestive system deals with food.

Cells

The structure of a typical cell

THE CELL MEMBRANE OR PLASMA MEMBRANE

This is the outer layer or boundary of the cell. It gives shape to the cell and protects it, separating things inside the cell (intracellular) from those outside the cell (extracellular). It regulates the passage of substances in and out of the cell.

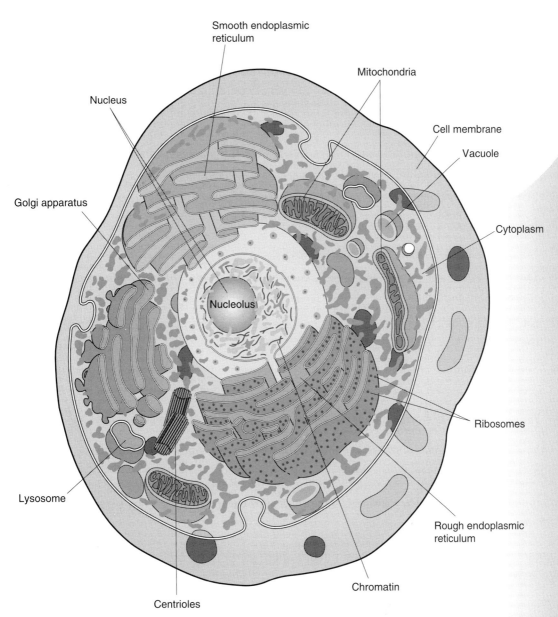

Figure 2.1   A typical cell.

THE CYTOPLASM

This is a soft jelly-like substance where the functions of the cell are carried out. It contains various structures called organelles (mini-organs), each of which has a specific function. Also in the cytoplasm are various chemical substances called inclusions.

THE ORGANELLES

These mini-organs each have a characteristic shape and role to perform. The type and number of organelles in different kinds of cell vary depending upon the activities of the cell, e.g. muscle cells have large numbers of mitochondria, because they have a high-level energy output.

◎ Nucleus – the largest of the organelles. It controls the activities of the cell and contains the body's genetic material (DNA)

◎ Mitochondria, which generate ATP/energy; there are large numbers in muscle cells

◎ Ribosomes, which synthesise protein

◎ Lysosomes, which digest and deal with waste

◎ The Golgi apparatus, which is concerned with the production of membrane and protein lipids and lipoproteins

◎ Endoplasmic reticulum – a series of channels for transporting substances within the cell

◎ The centrosome – involved in cell division.

THE INCLUSIONS

These are chemical substances produced by cells. They may not be present in all cells, e.g. melanin is a pigment found in certain cells of the skin and hair: it protects the body by screening out ultraviolet light, and gives the skin its brown colour on exposure to sunlight. Lipid (fat) is found in fat cells; this is broken down to provide energy when required.

Characteristics of cells are metabolism, respiration, growth, reproduction, excretion, irritability and movement.

Tissues

Groups of similar cells are organised together to form the body tissues. The cells of one tissue will all be the same, but they will be different for the different tissues. Tissues are classified into four types: epithelial, connective, muscular and nervous.

Table 2.1   Classification of tissues

Epithelial	Simple	Squamous – flat cells – lines heart, blood vessels, etc
		Cuboidal – cube shaped – lines ducts of glands
		Columnar – column shaped – lines stomach and body tracts
		Columnar ciliated – columns with hairs – lines respiratory tract
	Compound	Stratified squamous – layers of flat cells – lines mouth
		Cuboidal – ducts of sweat glands
		Columnar – lines male urethra and anus
		Transitional – lines bladder
	Glandular	Secreting cells found in glands

(*continued*)

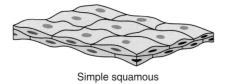

Simple squamous

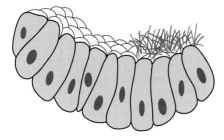

Cuboidal

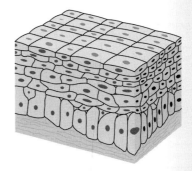

Stratified squamous

Simple columnar

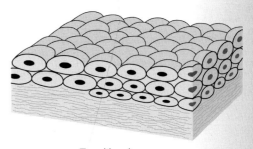

Transitional squamous

Figure 2.2   Types of epithelial tissue.

Table 2.1 (*continued*)

Connective tissue	Areolar	Connecting skin to tissues and muscles, lying around muscle bundles and binding muscles together
	Adipose	Stores fat under skin and around organs
	Dense fibrous	Gives tensile strength – ligaments and tendons
	Yellow elastic	Gives elasticity to skin and walls of arteries
	Reticular	Found in lymphatic tissue
	Cartilage	Fibro-cartilage – intervertebral discs
		Elastic cartilage – outer ear
		Hyaline cartilage – covers the ends of bones at joints
	Bone	Compact – outer layer of bones
		Cancellous – inner mass of bones
	Blood	Fluid connective tissue; transports substances around body and regulates body temperature
Muscular tissue	Skeletal	Produces body movement, maintains posture and produces heat
	Cardiac	Heart muscle maintains pumping action
	Smooth	Walls of blood vessels and intestines – peristalsis
Nervous tissue	Neurones	Pick up stimuli and conduct impulses to other neurones, muscle fibres or glands
	Neuroglia	Supporting substance that protects neurones

Membranes

There are four membranes that cover or line body parts:

1 Cutaneous: skin

2 Mucous: lines body tracts that open to exterior – respiratory and gastro-intestinal

3 Serous: lines body cavities, thorax and surrounds lungs

4 Synovial: lines joints up to the cartilage.

Body organs

Many tissues will be organised to form the organs of the body. Each organ has a specific function or functions to perform, e.g. the stomach digests food, lungs exchange gases, the heart pumps blood, kidneys form urine and filter fluids, and ovaries produce and release ova. Organs form parts of the systems of the body.

Body systems

Each body system consists of many organs that link together to perform a common function. All the systems are interrelated and function together to maintain life. There are 11 body systems (see table 2.2 overleaf):

- integumentary
- skeletal
- muscular
- nervous
- cardio-vascular
- lymphatic
- respiratory
- digestive
- urinary
- reproductive
- endocrine

❖ *The integumentary system* ❖

This system includes the skin, hair, nails, sweat and sebaceous glands and various sensory receptors that convey sensations to the spinal cord and brain.

Skin

The skin forms a tough, waterproof protective covering over the entire surface of the body; it is continuous with the membranes lining the orifices. It covers a surface area of approximately two square metres, and varies in thickness from 0.05 mm to 3 mm, being thickest on the soles of the feet and palms of the hands and thinnest on the lips, eyelids, inner surfaces of the limbs and on the abdomen. The skin includes hair, nails, glands and various sensory receptors.

Skin colour

Skin colour varies from person to person and from race to race. Skin colour is due to the pigment melanin, to the quantity of blood flowing through the blood vessels, and to the pigment carotene, which is present in the skin of certain races such as Asians. The number of melanocytes is approximately the same in all races, but colour varies because of the amount and type of melanin produced.

Healthy skin is smooth, soft and flexible and has a good colour. A grey, ashen or yellow tinge may indicate health problems.

Table 2.2   Classification of body systems

System	Structure	Function
Integumentary	The skin and all its structures – nails, hair, sweat and sebaceous glands	Protects, regulates temperature, eliminates waste, makes vitamin D, receives stimuli
Skeletal	The bones, joints and cartilages	Supports, protects, aids movement, stores fat and minerals, protects cells that produce blood cells
Muscular	Usually refers to skeletal muscle but includes cardiac and smooth	Produces movement, maintains posture and produces heat
Nervous	Brain, spinal cord, nerves and sense organs	Communicates and co-ordinates body functions
Cardio-vascular	Heart, blood vessels and blood	Transports substances around body, helps regulate body temperature and prevents blood loss by blood clotting
Lymphatic	Lymphatic vessels, nodes, ducts, lymph, spleen, tonsils and thymus gland	Returns proteins and plasma to blood. Carries fat from intestine to blood. Filters body fluid, forms white blood cells, fights infection and protects against disease
Respiratory	Pharynx, larynx, trachea, bronchi and lungs	Supplies oxygen and removes carbon dioxide
Digestive	Gastro-intestinal tract, salivary glands, gall bladder, liver and pancreas	Physical and chemical breakdown of food. Absorption of nutrients and elimination of waste
Urinary	Kidneys, ureters, bladder and urethra	Regulates chemical composition of blood. Helps to balance the acid/alkali content in the body and eliminates urine
Reproductive	All organs of reproduction – ovaries, testes, etc	Involved in reproduction and production of sex hormones
Endocrine	All the hormone-producing ductless glands	Hormones regulate a wide variety of body activities, e.g. growth, and maintain body balance (homeostasis)

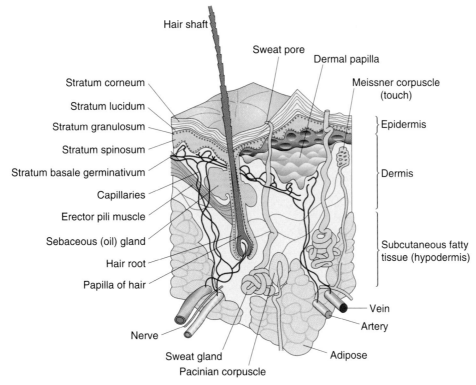

Figure 2.3   Cross-section through skin.

Skin structure

The skin is composed of two main layers with a subcutaneous fatty layer underneath. The two main layers are:

1   epidermis

2   dermis.

These layers may be further subdivided as follows:

1   The epidermis has five layers:
    a)   stratum corneum (superficial layer)
    b)   stratum lucidum
    c)   stratum granulosum
    d)   stratum spinosum
    e)   stratum basale (germinativum) (deepest layer).

2   The dermis has two layers:
    a)   papillary layer
    b)   reticular layer.

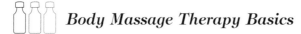

Epidermis

The epidermis is composed of **five layers** of stratified squamous epithelium. The living cells of the two deepest layers contain nuclei; the dead cells of the upper three layers lose their nuclei and become filled with a protein called **keratin**. As the cells of the stratum basale multiply they push upward, forming the next layer.

Stratum basale (Stratum germinativum)

This is the deepest layer of the epidermis. It is a single layer of cells on a basement membrane and lies directly on the papillary layer of the dermis. The capillary network of the dermis provides nutrients for these living cells.

The cells have a nucleus and multiply by mitosis (cell division).

Approximately one in ten of these basal cells are specialised cells called melanocytes. They produce the pigment melanin from the amino acid tyrosine.

Melanin is produced to protect the cells against the damaging effect of ultraviolet radiation. It gives the skin its brown colour.

This layer also contains the nerve endings sensitive to touch (Merkel's discs).

Stratum spinosum

This is composed of eight to ten layers of living cells. Granules of melanin pass into this layer.

The cells begin to lose their shape and have projections or spines, which join the cells together.

Stratum granulosum

This consists of three to five layers of flattened cells. Enzymes break down the nucleus and the cells die.

Keratohyaline is laid down in the cytoplasm, giving the first stages of keratinisation.

The protein keratin protects the skin from injury and invasion of micro-organisms and makes it waterproof.

Stratum lucidum

This is composed of several layers of clear, flat, dead cells that are translucent and filled with keratin.

This layer is found only on the palms of the hands and soles of the feet, where it provides extra protection.

Stratum corneum

This is the superficial layer, composed of many rows of flat, dead, scaly cells filled with keratin, which are constantly shed and replaced (this shedding of cells is known as desquamation).

Sebum secreted by the sebaceous glands helps to keep this layer soft and supple.

Rubbing or friction of the skin will increase the rate of desquamation.

Dermis

The dermis lies under the epidermis and is composed of two layers: the upper papillary layer and the lower reticular layer.

The surface of the papillary layer is ridged, forming an uneven surface. These finger-like projections increase the surface area and are called **dermal papillae**.

They produce the pattern known as finger prints. The blood capillary loops of the dermis transport nutrients and oxygen to basal layer cells and remove waste products. Some elastin and collagen fibres are found in the matrix.

The reticular layer is composed of dense irregular connective tissue with more collagen and elastin fibres. This gives the skin strength, extensibility and elasticity.

The skin's ability to stretch and recoil is necessary during pregnancy and obesity. The ground substance or matrix retains water, helping the skin to remain firm and turgid.

Many structures are found in the dermis. They include blood vessels, lymphatic vessels, sebaceous glands, sweat glands, nerves and nerve endings, hair in hair follicles, erector pili muscles, fibres (white fibres and yellow elastic fibres), fibroblasts, mast cells, plasma cells and macrophages.

Blood vessels

The dermis is well supplied with blood vessels, partly to provide nutrients to the actively dividing cells of the epidermis (which has no direct supply), but also to enable the skin to play its part in the regulation of body temperature. Small vessels leave the dermal plexus at right angles and pass upwards to the skin's surface, ending in the dermal papillae. Nutrients and oxygen pass out into the tissue fluid and into the basal cells, and waste products pass out of the cells into tissue fluid through capillaries to the small veins.

The amount of blood flowing near the surface of the skin is controlled by nerve endings in the artery walls. If the body is becoming too hot, the small arteries dilate (get bigger). This causes flushing of the skin known as **erythema** and the body loses heat via the skin. If the body becomes too cool the arteries constrict, preventing heat loss. Massage stimulates the nerve endings and by reflex action the blood vessels dilate producing an erythema.

Lymphatic vessels

There is a network of fine lymphatic capillaries and vessels throughout the dermis. They are blind-end tubes with walls of greater permeability than blood capillaries – larger particles can enter these vessels and be drained away in the lymph. The broken-down products of infection by micro-organisms are also drained away in the lymph.

Sebaceous glands

These glands secrete an oily substance called **sebum**. (It consists mainly of waxes, fats and fatty acids, and dehydrocholesterol, which forms vitamin D in sunlight.)

The glands are found in all areas except the soles and palms and between the fingers and toes. They are numerous on the scalp, forehead, nose, chin, chest and between the shoulders.

The glands are sac-like and are usually attached to the side wall of hair follicles into which the secretions enter via a duct, but some open directly onto the skin surface.

The glands are composed of epithelial cells that multiply, grow larger towards the centre and become filled with sebum. Eventually they burst, discharging sebum into the hair follicle.

The production of sebum is controlled by hormones (secreted by the endocrine glands). Hormonal imbalance, for example at puberty, increases the flow of sebum, often causing problems such as acne.

The function of the sebum is to coat the skin and hair and keep the surface smooth and supple.

It prevents loss of water from the skin.

It also has antiseptic and anti-fungal properties, protecting the skin from bacterial and fungal infections.

Sebum is gradually lost by washing and desquamation but is continually replaced. Massage stimulates the glands to produce more sebum.

Acid mantle

Together with the sweat secreted by sweat glands, sebum forms a coating on the skin known as the **acid mantle** because the secretions have a pH of between 4.5 and 6 (acidic). This is neutralised when the skin is washed with soap (alkali), but is restored if all the soap is rinsed away.

Sweat glands

There are two types of sweat gland:

1. **Eccrine glands** (sudoriferous): these consist of a coiled tube lying in the dermis with a straight duct opening in a pore on the skin surface. They are most numerous on the soles of feet and palms of hands.

2. **Apocrine glands** (odoriferous glands): these consist of coiled tubes larger than eccrine glands. They open into hair follicles, usually above the sebaceous glands. Sometimes they open directly onto the skin surface near a follicle. They are found in limited areas only, e.g. armpits and pubic areas.
   Development takes place at puberty. The secretion is somewhat viscous and sticky; when this is acted on by bacteria it leads to unpleasant body odour (BO).

Sweat

Sweat is a clear liquid containing 98% water, 2% sodium chloride and other substances, including urea and lactic acid. Sweat takes heat from the skin during evaporation. It therefore helps to maintain constant body temperature. Massage produces heat and therefore stimulates the sweat glands to produce more sweat.

Nerves

The skin is richly supplied with sensory nerve endings, which relay information about the environment to the nervous system. Most of the nerve endings lie in the dermis, but a few detecting pain lie in the lower layers of the epidermis. There are various types of nerve ending, modified according to their function. They detect cold, heat, pain and pressure (Meissner's corpuscles – touch; Merkel's discs – pressure; Pacinian corpuscles – vibration and deep pressure). These warn the body of harmful changes so that it can protect itself. The few motor nerves control secretion of sweat and contraction of erector pili muscles. These nerve endings may be soothed by massage, but if the massage is too light they may be irritated and if it is too deep, pain is increased. These factors will increase tension and must be avoided.

Hair

Hairs are dead, horny structures composed of keratinised cells. They are found all over the body except on the soles and palms. They vary in length, texture and colour. Hairs are embedded in a depression called a hair follicle. The hair follicle consists of epithelial cells that form a tube passing obliquely into the dermis. It encases the hair bulb and hair root. The hair bulb is the expanded part of the hair that lies at the base of the follicle in the dermis. The hair root grows from the bulb and up through the follicle to the skin's surface. The hair shaft is the part that extends beyond the surface of the skin. Massage is more comfortable if it is performed in the direction of the hair growth, but this is not always possible.

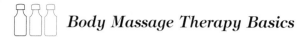

Erector pili muscles

These are small involuntary muscles connected to the hair follicles. When they contract they pull the hair follicles straight. This happens during extreme fright or cold – the skin around the follicle becomes raised, forming 'goose flesh'.

Fibres

These consist of white collagen fibres and yellow elastic fibres.

White fibres are formed from non-elastic fibres of the protein collagen, lying in layers. They give the skin tensile strength and flexibility, and they bind structures together.

Yellow elastic fibres are formed from the protein elastin. They are scattered throughout the matrix. These highly elastic fibres are capable of stretch and recoil. They give the skin elasticity, enabling it to stretch and return to normal. This is important for pregnancy and obesity. If the skin is over-stretched small tears occur in the dermis. These can be seen as white lines called 'stretch marks'. With ageing, the skin loses elasticity and becomes wrinkled. Care must be taken when massaging older clients not to further stretch the skin. All fibres are embedded in a jelly-like matrix. This is capable of absorbing water, giving firmness to the skin.

Cells

1. Fibroblasts produce the matrix and fibres.

2. Mast cells release **histamine** following injury or reaction to an allergen. Histamine initiates an inflammatory response, causing dilation of capillaries and increasing the permeability of cell walls. This process aids tissue repair.

3. Plasma cells produce antibodies.

4. Leucocytes destroy, and protect the body against, micro-organisms.

5. Macrophages clean up cellular debris.

Functions of the skin

Sensitivity   The skin contains many sensory receptors, which register changes in the external environment. These receptors are sensitive to touch, pressure, pain, heat and cold. From the nerve endings in the skin, impulses are transmitted to the brain where an appropriate response is initiated.

Heat regulation   The skin is one of the main organs for body temperature control. Normal body temperature is 37°C or 98.4°F. Heat regulation is achieved by:

◎   evaporation of sweat: body heat is used for the evaporation of sweat; this lowers body temperature.

◎   dilation and constriction of blood capillaries in the skin: if the body becomes too hot, the surface capillaries dilate and more blood flows to the surface, giving off heat. When this happens the skin becomes pink or red; this reddening of the skin is known as *erythema*. If the body becomes too cold the blood vessels constrict and less blood flows to the surface. Therefore less heat is lost and body temperature is maintained.

◎   insulation by adipose tissue: the fatty tissue in the dermis and subcutaneous layer acts as an insulating layer that helps to retain body heat.

Absorption   The absorption of substances through the skin is limited. The keratin in the cells and the covering of sebum prevent the absorption of water, making the skin waterproof. However, the skin will allow certain substances to pass through so that drugs, hormones and other substances are sometimes administered through the skin.

Protection   This is a very important function. The skin forms an effective barrier, which protects the body from harm. The skin gives protection from:

◎   *Dirt and chemical attack*, the keratin and flat dead cells in the superficial layers of the skin protect against dirt and chemical attack.

◎   *Invasion by micro-organisms*, the mixture of sebum and sweat forms an acid mantle over the surface of the skin. The pH of the skin is around 5 and this slightly acidic environment discourages the growth of micro-organisms.

◎   *Minor injuries*, through the sensory nerve endings in the skin the brain can quickly respond to painful stimuli thus protecting the body from damage.

◎   *UV radiation*, the melanocytes (cells that produce melanin) in the stratum germinativum produce the pigment melanin, which protects the underlying tissues from the harmful effects of ultra-violet rays.

Excretion   The skin plays a minor role in the excretion of urea and other waste products through sweating.

Secretion and storage   The sebaceous glands secrete sebum, which, with sweat, forms the protective acid mantle. Sebum also lubricates the skin, keeping it soft and supple. The skin stores water and fat.

Formation of vitamin D   This is an important function of the skin. It forms vitamin D from the action of sunlight on the chemical 7 dehydrocholesterol in the skin.

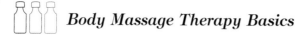

Effects of massage on the skin

◎ Massage improves the condition of the skin because the increased blood supply increases the delivery of nutrients and oxygen and speeds up the removal of metabolic waste. Metabolism is increased, which stimulates the cells of the stratum basale and increases mitosis (cell division). More cells move upwards towards the surface, improving the condition of the skin as old cells are replaced.

◎ Massage aids desquamation (shedding of dead cells). Increased mitosis will increase the shedding of the flaky dead cells of the stratum corneum. Also, the friction of the hands on the skin will rub off these dead cells on the surface.

◎ The colour of the skin is improved. Massage produces dilation of surface capillaries: this results in hyperaemia and erythema, which improve the colour of sallow skin.

◎ Sebaceous glands are stimulated to produce and release more sebum. This lubricates the skin and keeps it soft and supple.

◎ The oil or cream used as a medium also lubricates and softens the skin.

◎ Sweat glands are stimulated to produce more sweat, which aids cleansing and elimination of waste.

Effects of massage on adipose tissue

Adipose tissue is a connective tissue composed mainly of specialised cells called adipocytes, adapted to store fat. It is found under the skin in the subcutaneous layer and around organs. Fat is the body's energy reserve. It is *stored* when energy intake is greater than energy output and *utilised* if energy intake is less than energy output. Therefore, the only way of losing fat is through sensible eating and increasing activity or exercise. However, massage is thought to help the dispersal of fat because the deeper movements stimulate blood flow to the area. This softens the area and may speed up removal via the circulating blood from that area, providing the client also reduces intake of food.

The effects of massage on cellulite (very hard consolidated fat) is dealt with in Chapter 8.

❖ *The skeletal system* ❖

The skeletal system is made up of bones, joints and cartilages. The human skeleton is made up of 206 bones. These are grouped into two main divisions: the **axial skeleton**, which forms the core or axis of the body, and the **appendicular skeleton**, which forms the girdles and limbs. It is important to identify skeletal bones, particularly those with bony points or prominences, which must be avoided when massaging.

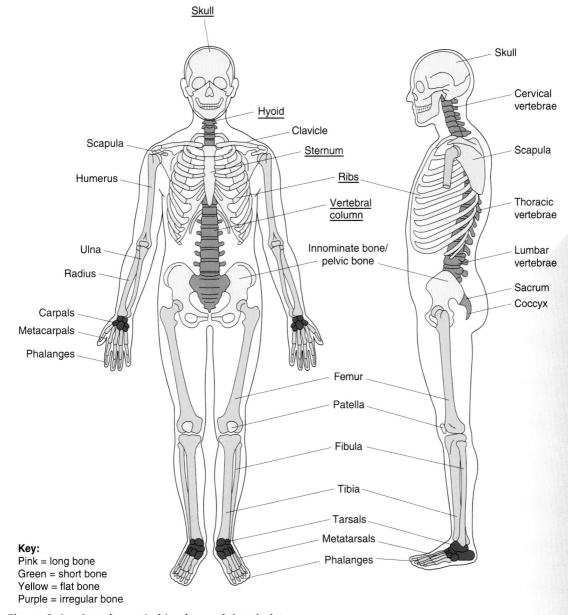

Figure 2.4   Anterior and side views of the skeleton.

The axial skeleton

The bones of the axial skeleton include the:

◎   skull (the cranium and bones of the face)

◎   vertebral column (spine)

◎   sternum (breast bone)

- ribs
- hyoid bone (small bone in neck below mandible).

Appendicular skeleton

The bones of the appendicular skeleton include the:

UPPER LIMB

- clavicle (collar bone)
- scapula (shoulder bone)
- humerus (upper arm bone)
- radius (forearm – lateral)
- ulna (forearm – medial)
- carpals (wrist)
- metacarpals (palm)
- phalanges (fingers).

LOWER LIMB

- innominate or pelvic bone (hip bone)
- femur (thigh bone)
- patella (knee cap)
- tibia (large bone of lower leg – medial)
- fibula (thin bone of lower leg – lateral)
- tarsals (ankle)
- metatarsals (foot)
- phalanges (toes).

Vertebral column

The vertebral column (also known as the spinal column) is composed of 33 vertebrae. Some are fused together, making 26 bones. The vertebrae are separated by intervertebral discs of fibro-cartilage, which act as shock absorbers. The bones and discs are bound together by strong ligaments.

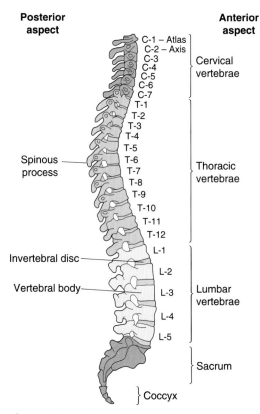

Figure 2.5 The vertebral column.

The column is divided into five regions:

1	**cervical**	7 vertebrae (neck), concave when viewed posteriorly
2	**thoracic**	12 vertebrae (upper back), convex when viewed posteriorly
3	**lumbar**	5 vertebrae (lower, small of back), concave when viewed posteriorly
4	**sacral**	5 fused vertebrae (sacrum), convex when viewed posteriorly
5	**coccygeal**	4 fused vertebrae (coccyx).

The functions of the skeleton

1 Support – the bony framework gives shape to the body, supports the soft tissues and provides attachments for muscles.

2 Protection – the bony framework protects delicate internal organs from injury, e.g. the brain is protected by the skull; the heart and lungs are protected by the rib cage.

3 Movement – produced by a system of bones, joints and muscles. The bones act as levers, and muscles pull on the bones, resulting in movement at the joints.

4 Storage of minerals – bones store many minerals, particularly calcium and phosphorus.

5 Storage of energy – fats or lipids stored in the yellow bone marrow provide energy when required.

6 Storage of tissue that forms blood cells – both red and white blood cells are produced by red bone marrow, which is found in the spongy bone of the pelvis, vertebrae, ribs, sternum and in the ends of the femur and humerus.

Joints

A joint is where two or more bones join or articulate. There are three main groups: fibrous, cartilaginous and synovial.

Types of joint

1 **Fibrous**: immoveable joints; the bones fit tightly together and are held firmly by fibrous tissue. There is no joint cavity. Examples are the sutures of the skull.

2 **Cartilaginous**: slightly moveable joints; the bones are connected by a disc or plate of fibro-cartilage. There is no joint cavity. Examples are the symphysis pubis (between the pubic bones) and the intervertebral joints (between the vertebral bodies).

3 **Synovial**: freely moveable joints; these are the most numerous in the body. There are six different types of synovial joint. They are classified according to their planes of

movement, which depend on the shape of the articulating bones. All the freely moveable joints of the body are synovial joints and, although their shape and movements vary, they all have certain characteristics in common:

a) a **joint cavity** (space within the joint)

b) a **synovial membrane** lining the capsule of the joint up to the hyaline cartilage, which produces synovial fluid

c) **synovial fluid** or synovium – a viscous fluid that lubricates and nourishes the joint

d) **hyaline cartilage**, which covers the surfaces of the articulating bones. It is sometimes called articular cartilage. It reduces friction and allows smooth movement

e) a **capsule**, or articulating capsule, which surrounds the joints like a sleeve. It holds the bones together and encloses the cavity. The capsule is strengthened on the outside by ligaments, which help to stabilise and strengthen the joints. Ligaments may also be found inside a joint, holding bones together and increasing stability. Massage is used around joints to increase the circulation and to free ligaments that may have become bound down following injury.

Discs (menisci)

Some joints have pads of fibro-cartilage called discs. They are attached to the bones and give the joint a better 'fit'. They also cushion movement, e.g. cartilages of the knee.

Bursae

Any movement produces friction between the moving parts. In order to reduce friction, sac-like structures containing synovial fluid are found between tissues. These are called bursae and are usually found between tendons and bone.

Classification or types of the six synovial joints

1. **gliding joint**, e.g. intercarpal or intertarsal joints

2. **hinge joint**, e.g. elbow or knee

3. **pivot joint**, e.g. superior radio-ulnar joint or atlas on axis

4. **ellipsoid joint** (condyloid), e.g. wrist or knuckle joints

5. **saddle joint**, e.g. base of the thumb

6. **ball-and-socket joint**, shoulder or hip joint

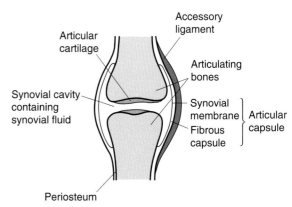

Figure 2.6a   A synovial joint.

Although synovial joints differ in shape and movement range,
they all have similar characteristics

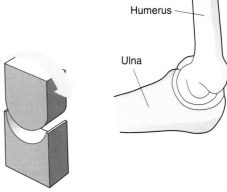

Humerus

Ulna

A ball and socket joint: found in the shoulder and the hip. Designed to allow a wide range of movement

A hinge joint: found at the elbow and knee. The range of movement is limited to one plane, such as a door hinge

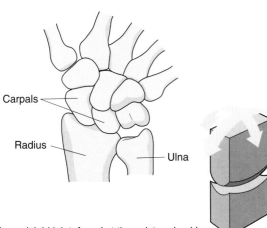

Carpals

Radius

Ulna

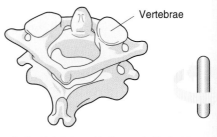

Vertebrae

A condyloid joint: found at the wrist and ankle. Movement in two planes, but not such a full range as in the ball and socket joint

A pivot joint: found in the neck. Part of the bone fits into another ring of bone as in atlas and axis, allowing rotation of the head

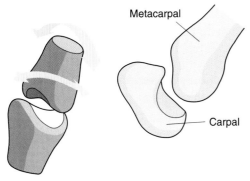

Metacarpal

Carpal

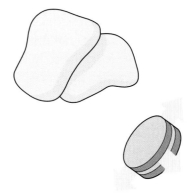

A saddle joint: found at the base of the thumb. This joint allows the thumb to be moved in two directions and circled around

A gliding joint: found in the wrist between the carpal bones. Two bones have a small range of gliding movement limited by connecting ligaments

Figure 2.6b Types of synovial joint.

Effects of massage on bone tissue and joints

◎ Bones are covered by a layer of connective tissue known as the 'periosteum'. Blood vessels from the periosteum penetrate the bone. Deep massage movements will stimulate blood flow to the periosteum and hence indirectly increase blood supply to the bone.

◎ Massage around joints will increase the circulation and nourish the structures surrounding the joint.

◎ Massage is effective in loosening adhesions in structures around joints. For example, frictions across a ligament help to loosen it from underlying structures.

◎ Massage and passive movements will help to maintain full range of movement.

❖ *The muscular system* ❖

There are three types of muscle tissue:

1 Skeletal muscle – forms the body flesh and produces body movement

2 Cardiac muscle – forms the walls of the heart and pumps blood around the body

3 Smooth muscle – found in the walls of the intestines (viscera), which contract to move food along in the digestive tract (peristalsis).

Skeletal muscle forms the body flesh. The function of skeletal muscle is to produce movement, maintain posture and produce body heat. Skeletal muscle tissue is totally under the control of the nervous system; impulses transmitted from the brain via motor nerves initiate contraction of muscle fibres. This muscle contraction pulls on bones and movement occurs at joints.

Structure of skeletal muscle

Skeletal muscle is composed of muscle fibres arranged in bundles called **fasciculi**. Many bundles of fibres make up the complete muscle. The fibres, bundles and muscles are surrounded and protected by connective tissue sheaths.

Skeletal muscle fibres are long, thin multi-nucleated cells. These fibres are made up of even smaller protein threads called myofibrils. These run the whole length of the fibre and are the elements that contract and relax. Each myofibril is composed of actin and myosin protein threads that slide into each other so that the myofibril shortens. When these myofibrils shorten, the whole muscle contracts.

◎ The connective tissue around each fibre is called the **endomysium**.

◎ The connective tissue around each bundle is called the **perimysium**.

◎ The connective tissue around the muscle is called the **epimysium**.

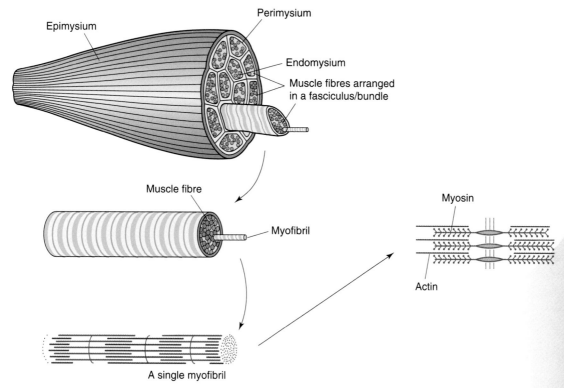

Figure 2.7   Construction of skeletal muscle.

If this connective tissue becomes tight or adheres to underlying structures, the muscle function is impaired. The petrissage movements and myofascial stretching techniques are very effective in freeing and stretching the tissue, allowing the muscle fibres to function normally.

Muscle fibres

Muscle fibres are long, thin, multi-nucleated cells. The fibres vary from 10 to 100 microns in diameter, and from a few millimetres to many centimetres in length. The long fibres extend the full length of the muscle while the short fibres end in connective tissue intersections within the muscle.

Muscle attachments

As previously explained, a muscle is composed of muscle fibres and connective tissue components – the endomysium, perimysium and epimysium. Certain muscles have connective tissue intersections dividing the muscle into several bellies, as seen in *rectus abdominis*.

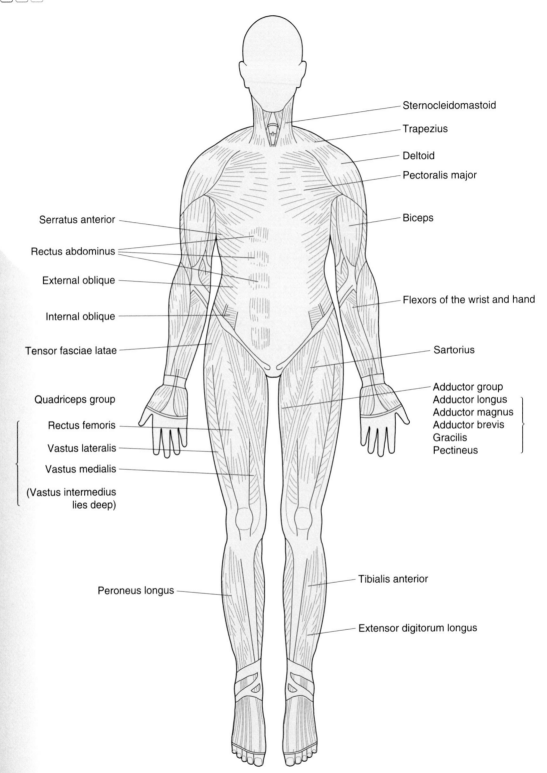

Figure 2.8a   Muscles of the body – anterior.

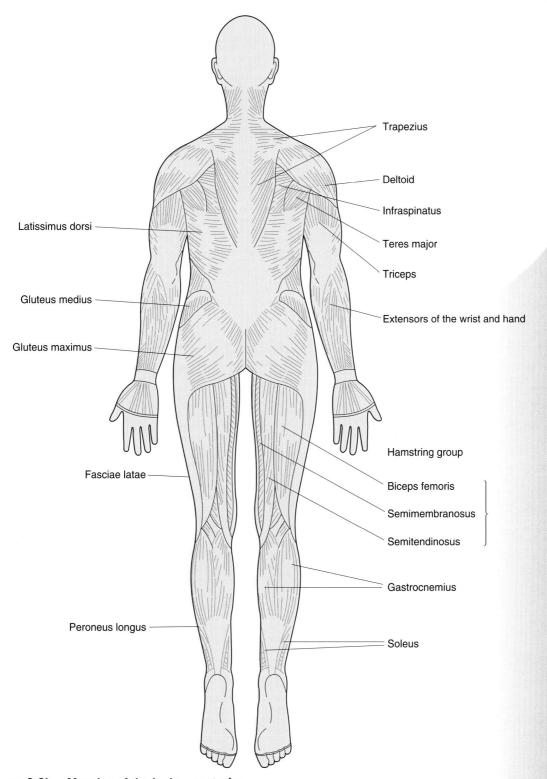

Trapezius

Deltoid

Infraspinatus

Teres major

Triceps

Extensors of the wrist and hand

Latissimus dorsi

Gluteus medius

Gluteus maximus

Hamstring group

Biceps femoris

Semimembranosus

Semitendinosus

Gastrocnemius

Fasciae latae

Peroneus longus

Soleus

Figure 2.8b   Muscles of the body – posterior.

These sheets of connective tissue blend at either end of the muscle and attach the muscle to underlying bones. Muscles are attached via tendons or aponeuroses.

◎ **Tendons** are tough cord-like structures of connective tissue that attach muscles to bones.

◎ **Aponeuroses** are flat sheets of connective tissue that attach muscles along the length of bone.

A muscle has at least two points of attachment, known as the origin and insertion of the muscle.

◎ The **origin** is usually proximal and stationary or immoveable.

◎ The **insertion** is usually distal and moveable.

Following over-use or injury, these tendons may become inflamed. Massage around the area can restore function. Transverse frictions are useful for freeing tendons held by adhesions.

Muscle shape

Muscle shape varies depending on the function of the muscle. The fleshy bulk of the muscle is known as the belly. The muscle fibres forming bundles lie parallel or obliquely to the line of pull of the muscle. Parallel fibres are found in strap-like and fusiform muscles. These long fibres allow for a wide range of movement. Oblique fibres are found in triangular and pennate muscles. These shorter fibres are found where muscle strength is required.

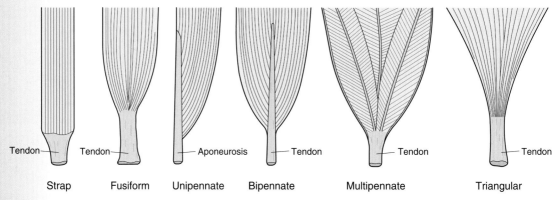

Figure 2.9   Muscle shapes.

Blood supply to skeletal muscle

Supplies of oxygen and nutrients required by muscles to produce energy for muscle contraction are transported in the blood via the arteries supplying the muscle; the waste products are removed via the veins. The arteries branch to form smaller arteries and arterioles within the perimysium. They then further divide forming capillary networks within the endomysium, where they join venules that lead to veins. When muscles are relaxed, the capillary network delivers blood to the muscle fibres. When muscles contract, the pressure impedes the flow of blood through the capillary beds, which reduces the supply of oxygen and nutrients and limits removal of waste. During exercise, muscle fibres alternately contract and relax, and the capillaries deliver blood during the relaxation phase. However, repeated or sustained contractions, such as isometric work or exercising without sufficient rest periods, prevents blood flow to the muscle fibres, due to compression on blood vessels and capillaries. This results in **muscle fatigue**, due to lack of oxygen and nutrients and the accumulation of waste products such as lactic acid. The strength and speed of contraction becomes progressively weaker until the muscle finally fails to relax completely, resulting in muscle spasm and pain.

Long effleurage strokes speed up venous return and the circulation to the muscle is increased. Accumulated waste is removed and pain and stiffness relieved. The squeezing movements of petrissage also increase the circulation. When tension in the muscle is relieved, pressure is decreased and circulation flows normally through the capillary beds.

Muscle tone

Muscle tone is the state of partial contraction or tension found in muscles even when at rest. Only a small number of muscle fibres will be in a state of contraction. This is sufficient to produce tautness in the muscle but not to result in full contraction and movement. Different groups of fibres contract alternately, working a 'shift' system to prevent fatigue. Changes in muscle tone are adjusted according to the information received from sensory receptors within the muscles and their tendons. **Muscle spindles** transmit information on the degree of stretch within the muscle. **Tendon receptors** called Golgi organs transmit information on the amount of tension applied to the tendon by muscle contraction. Too much stretch and tension will result in reduction in muscle tone. Too little will result in increase in muscle tone. Muscle tone is essential for maintaining upright postures.

◎ Hypotonic muscles, i.e. those with less than the normal degree of tone, are said to be **flaccid**.

◎ Hypertonic muscles, i.e. those with greater than normal degree of tone, are said to be **spastic**.

Effects of massage on muscle tissue

◎ Massage aids the relaxation of muscles, due to the warmth created, reflex response and removal of accumulated waste.

◎ Massage pushes the blood along in the veins. Deoxygenated blood and waste are removed and fresh oxygenated blood and nutrients are brought to the muscles. The metabolic rate is increased and the condition of the muscles will improve.

◎ Massage will reduce pain, stiffness and muscle fatigue produced by the accumulation of waste following anaerobic contraction. The removal of this metabolic waste, i.e. lactic acid and carbon dioxide, is speeded up and normal function is more quickly restored. This is particularly important following hard training, sport and athletic performance, for example, when massage will speed up the recovery of muscles, allowing the athlete to return to training more quickly. The increased nutrients and oxygen will also facilitate tissue repair and recovery.

◎ Massage warms muscles due to the increased blood flow, the friction of the hands moving over the area and the friction of the tissues as they move over each other. This reduces tension and aids relaxation of the muscles. Warm muscles contract more efficiently and are more extensile than cold muscles. Thus performance is enhanced and the likelihood of strains, sprains, micro-tears or other injury is reduced. Massage prior to exercise must be used in conjunction with (but not instead of) warm-up and stretch exercise.

◎ The elasticity of muscles is improved because manipulations such as kneading, wringing and picking up, stretch the fibres and separate the bundles. Any restricting fibrous adhesions are broken down and any tight fascia surrounding the bundles are stretched, allowing muscle fibres to function normally.

◎ Massage will break down adhesions and fibrositic nodules that may have developed within the muscle as a result of tension, poor posture or injury.

❖ *The cardio-vascular system* ❖

The cardio-vascular (blood circulatory) system is a closed circuit. It is composed of a pump called the heart, a network of interconnecting tubes called blood vessels, and the fluid flowing through the circuit known as blood. The parts that make up the system are:

➤ heart

➤ arteries and arterioles

➤ veins and venules

➤ capillaries

➤ blood.

The system is designed to carry blood to and from the organs and cells of the body. Blood carries oxygen, nutrients, hormones and enzymes to the cells, and takes away the waste products of metabolism from the cells.

Tissue fluid

All body cells are bathed in interstitial fluid (tissue fluid). This fluid provides a medium for substances to move across from the blood to the cells and from the cells to the blood.

Oxygenated blood flows from the heart, through the arteries and arterioles, and into the capillaries.

The walls of the capillaries are very thin: consequently the oxygen and nutrients pass out through the walls into the tissue fluid and from there into the cells.

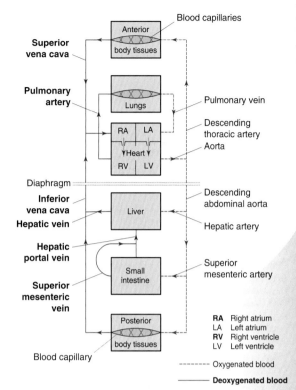

Figure 2.10   Circulation of blood.

The waste products of metabolism pass out of the cells into the tissue fluid and into the capillaries in the same way. This deoxygenated blood is transported via the venules and veins back to the heart.

The heart then pumps it to the lungs to be reoxygenated.

Some fluid and larger particles of waste are removed from the tissues via the thinner-walled lymphatic vessels. These lie alongside blood vessels among the tissues.

The heart

The heart lies in the thoracic cavity between the lungs. It is somewhat cone shaped, with the base above and the apex below. The walls of the heart are made up of three layers:

1. **pericardium**: a tough outer coat of fibrous tissue

2. **myocardium**: the middle coat of cardiac muscle

3. **endocardium**: the inner lining of squamous epithelium.

The heart is divided into a right and left side by a muscular wall or septum. The left side of the heart deals with **oxygenated** blood. The right side deals with **deoxygenated** blood. Each side is further divided into two chambers separated by valves. The upper chambers are called **atria** (singular: atrium); the lower chambers are called **ventricles**.

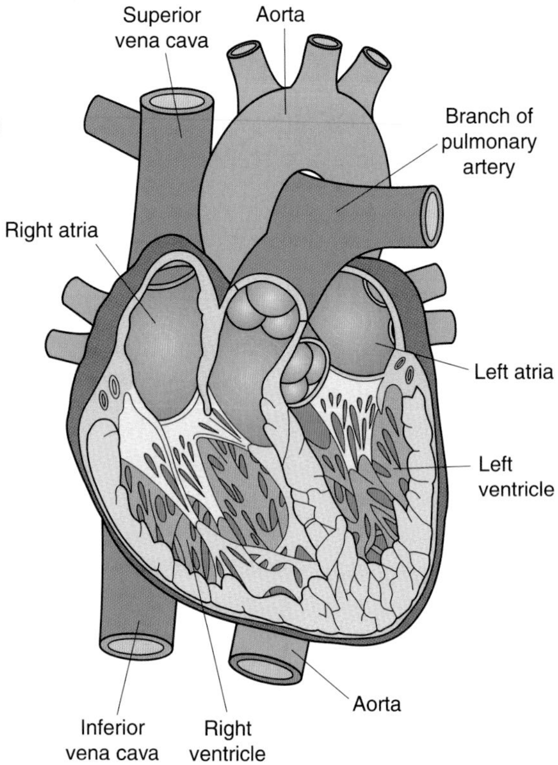

Flow of blood through the heart

◎ The inferior and superior venae cavae (veins) collect deoxygenated blood from the body and empty it into the right atrium.

◎ This blood then passes through the tricuspid valve into the right ventricle.

◎ From the right ventricle it is pumped into the pulmonary artery (the only artery carrying deoxygenated blood) and carried to the lungs.

◎ Interchange of gases occurs in the lungs and the oxygenated blood is carried by the pulmonary vein (the only vein carrying oxygenated blood) back to the left atrium of the heart.

◎ This blood passes through the bicuspid valve into the left ventricle.

◎ From the left ventricle, blood is pumped into the aorta – the first artery of the general circulation. The aorta branches into numerous arteries, which carry oxygenated blood to all body parts.

Figure 2.11   The heart.

Blood vessels

There are three main types of blood vessel: arteries, veins and capillaries.

Arteries transport oxygenated blood from the heart around the body to all tissues and organs. The main artery, the large *aorta*, leaves the left ventricle of the heart and divides to form other arteries, which further subdivide forming a network of arteries all over the body. Arteries finally divide into small thinly-walled vessels called arterioles, which enter the capillary networks among the tissues. Arteries transport blood carrying oxygen, nutrients, hormones etc around the body. Artery walls have three layers of tissues: a fibrous outer layer, a muscular middle layer and an inner lining of smooth epithelium. The middle muscular layer of arteries is thicker than the muscular layer of veins and their lumen is smaller. Blood is pumped through the

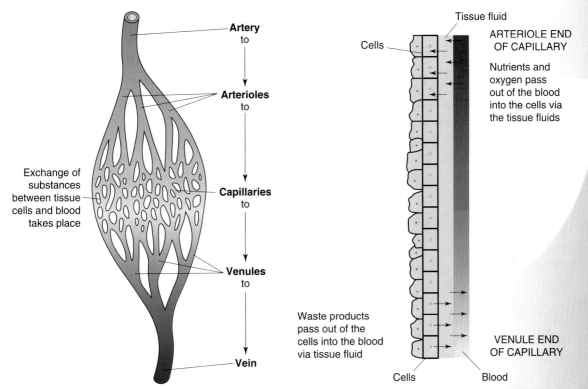

Figure 2.12a   Blood flow from artery to vein.

Figure 2.12b   Transfer of substances between the blood and cells.

arteries, around the body, by the contraction of the heart; with each contraction the blood is forced along. The rate at which the heart is beating can be felt as a pulse at arteries that lie near the surface, such as the radial artery at the wrist.

Veins transport deoxygenated blood back to the heart. The walls are similar in structure to those of arteries but the middle muscular layer is thinner. The inner layer of epithelial cells is folded to form valves. These valves prevent the backward flow of blood. The lumen of veins is larger than that of arteries.

Blood is pumped along the veins by the contraction and relaxation of muscles and by the expansion and contraction of the thorax and diaphragm during breathing. If muscles are not contracting, e.g. during long periods of standing and inactivity, gravity exerts a downward force. If the valves are weak, blood 'pools' in the veins. This pressure overloads the veins and the wall bulges outwards, causing the condition known as varicose veins. Regular leg massage speeds up the flow of blood through the veins. This prevents overloading of the veins, which helps prevent varicose veins.

During periods of prolonged inactivity such as bed rest or sitting in cramped conditions for a long time, the flow of blood through the veins slows down and there is a risk of blood clots forming in the veins. A clot may attach to the vessel wall where it is called a **thrombus** or it may become detached and be carried in the bloodstream, where it is known as an **embolus**. The clot may end up blocking the blood supply to the lung with potentially fatal consequences. This is one of the greatest dangers of massage, making thrombosis an absolute contra-indication to massage (see page 116).

Capillaries are thin-walled, tiny vessels that form networks among the tissue spaces. Arterioles enter capillary networks and venules leave. The primary function of capillaries is to allow the exchange of gases, nutrients and metabolic waste between the cells and the blood. Arterioles bring oxygen and nutrients to the capillaries. These pass through the thin vessel walls into the tissue fluid and then through the cell wall into the cell. Carbon dioxide and metabolites pass out of the cell and into the blood in the same way.

Venules leave the capillary networks and join to form larger veins that transport the deoxygenated blood and the waste products of metabolism (metabolites) back to the heart via the largest veins, namely the *inferior vena cava* and the *superior vena cava*. These two large veins empty into the right atrium of the heart.

When the metabolic needs of the tissues are low, parts of the capillary network can shut off, limiting blood flow. More blood is then available for those tissues with greater metabolic needs. Thus blood flow can be shunted in this way to areas that require a greater supply of oxygen and nutrients, e.g. exercising muscles.

Massage aids the dilation of these surface capillaries by reflex action, promoting blood flow. An accumulation of waste products in the tissues, or tension in muscle fibres, exerts pressure on the capillaries and restricts blood flow. Massage helps to relieve this pressure, as it speeds up the removal of waste products and promotes muscle relaxation. Thus the pressure is reduced and normal blood flow through the capillaries is restored. This helps the recovery of the muscles and restores normal function.

Blood

Blood is a viscous fluid (slightly sticky) that flows through the heart and blood vessels. It is composed of 55% plasma and 45% cells. (Plasma is a faintly yellow transparent fluid composed of 91% water, 7% proteins and 2% other solutes.) Its temperature is around 38°C and its pH is around 7.4 (slightly alkaline). The total volume of blood in the human body is 5–6 litres in men and 4–5 litres in women.

Blood cells

There are three main types of blood cell:

1. **erythrocytes**: red blood cells, which contain haemoglobin that transports oxygen and carbon dioxide

2 | **leucocytes**: white blood cells, which protect the body against invading micro-organisms; they play a part in the body's defence system and immune reaction

3 | **thrombocytes** or **platelets**: they play an important role in blood clotting.

Functions of the blood

1 | It **transports**

- ◎ oxygen from the lungs to body cells
- ◎ carbon dioxide from the cells to the lungs
- ◎ nutrients from the digestive tract to body cells
- ◎ metabolic waste products from cells to excretory organs
- ◎ hormones from endocrine glands to cells
- ◎ any drugs taken for medicinal purposes.

2 | It **regulates**

- ◎ the water content of cells
- ◎ body heat, maintaining normal body temperature
- ◎ pH by means of buffers.

3 | It **protects**

- ◎ against disease and infection, by the action of leucocytes, which destroy micro-organisms through phagocytic action and production of antibodies
- ◎ against blood loss by the process of blood clotting.

Blood pressure

This is the force or pressure the blood exerts on the walls of the blood vessels. The blood pressure in arteries is higher than that in veins. Blood pressure varies with sex, age and weight, and with activities, stress levels or anxiety. The condition of the heart and vessels also affects pressure.

Normal average blood pressure rises to around 120 mmHg (millimetres of mercury) as the heart contracts (systolic pressure), and falls to around 80 mmHg as the heart relaxes (diastolic pressure). Blood pressure is measured using a **sphygmomanometer** and expressed

as $BP = \dfrac{120}{80}$ mmHg.

Pulse

The pulse rate is the same as the heart rate, being around 74 beats per minute. The pulse can be felt in arteries because of the expansion and recoil of their walls during each ventricular contraction of the heart. The pulse is strongest in the arteries closest to the heart. The pulse is usually taken at the radial artery at the wrist, but can also be taken at the carotid artery in the neck and the brachial artery in the arm, medial to the biceps muscle.

Effects of massage on blood circulation

◎ Massage is thought to increase the blood flow through the area being treated, i.e. it produces hyperaemia (increased blood supply) and erythema (reddening of the skin).

◎ It speeds up the flow of blood through the veins. Veins lie superficially (nearer the surface than arteries). As the hands move over the part in the direction of venous return, the blood is pushed along in the veins towards the heart. The deeper and faster the movements, the greater the flow. This venous blood carries away metabolic waste products more quickly. If these are allowed to accumulate in muscle tissue they produce pain and stiffness, and exert pressure, which further restricts the circulation. Therefore, massage will relieve pain and stiffness by flushing out metabolic waste and relieving pressure on the capillaries, which restores free flow of blood within the tissues.

◎ It increases the supply of fresh, oxygenated blood to the part. As the deoxygenated blood is moved along, the capillaries empty and fresh oxygenated blood flows into them more quickly. The nutrients and oxygen nourish the tissues and aid tissue recovery and repair.

◎ Massage dilates superficial arterioles and capillaries, which improves the exchange of substances in and out of cells via tissue fluid. This will improve the metabolic rate, which, in turn, will improve the condition of the tissues. This dilation of the superficial capillaries produces an erythema (redness of the skin).

◎ Warmth is produced in the area due to the increased blood flow and friction of the hands on the part.

◎ Massage is thought to reduce the viscosity of the blood, reducing its rate of coagulation.

◎ Relaxing slow massage may reduce high blood pressure.

❖ *The lymphatic system* ❖

The lymphatic system is closely associated with the cardio-vascular system and connects with it. The lymphatic system removes tissue fluid and proteins from the tissue spaces and returns it to the blood via the subclavian veins. This fluid in the lymphatic vessels is called **lymph**. The system also transports fats from the small intestine to the blood, and it plays an important role in protecting the body against infection.

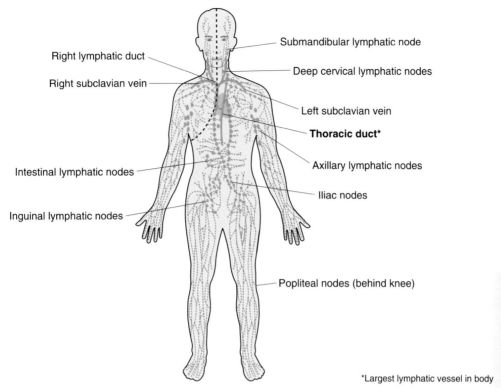

Figure 2.13   The lymphatic system.

The parts of the lymphatic system are:

➤ lymphatic capillaries, vessels and trunks: these are tubes that carry the fluid

➤ lymphatic nodes: arranged in groups throughout the body

➤ lymphatic organs: such as the spleen, thymus gland and tonsils

➤ lymphatic ducts: there are two ducts, the right lymphatic duct and the thoracic duct, which empty into the right and left subclavian veins

➤ lymph: the fluid flowing through the vessels.

Lymphatic capillaries begin as blind-end tubes forming a network among the tissue spaces. Their walls are very thin and allow fluid, larger proteins and particles to pass through. Because these larger particles and proteins are unable to pass through blood vessel walls, they are returned to the blood via the lymphatic system. These minute lymphatic capillaries then join together to form larger lymphatic vessels. Lymphatic vessels are very similar to veins in structure, but have thinner walls and a greater number of valves to prevent backward flow.

All lymphatic vessels drain into lymphatic nodes. These are strategically placed in groups along the path of the vessels. Many afferent vessels enter a node, but only one or two efferent vessels

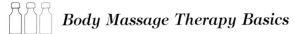

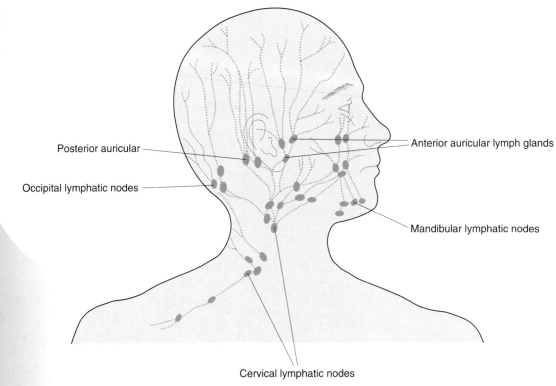

Figure 2.14 The lymphatic system of the head.

leave. Lymphatic nodes are small, bean-shaped structures up to 2 cm in length. Here the lymph is filtered, foreign substances are trapped and destroyed, and lymphocytes are produced that combat infection and disease. The efferent vessels leaving the nodes join to form lymphatic trunks. These empty into two main ducts:

1 **thoracic duct**: this receives lymph from the left arm, left side of the head and chest and all the body below the ribs; it empties into the left subclavian vein

2 **right lymphatic duct**: this receives lymph from the right upper quarter of the body, i.e. the right arm, right side of head and chest; it then empties into the right subclavian vein.

In this way the lymph is transported from the tissue spaces back to the blood. Any malfunction or blockage of the lymphatic system will result in swelling of the tissues known as **oedema.**

The speed at which lymph flows through the system depends on many factors, for example the contraction and relaxation of muscles help its return, as do negative pressure and movement of the chest during respiration. Exercise is therefore very important in aiding the flow of lymph. Areas of stasis and oedema can be improved by moving the joints and exercising the muscles

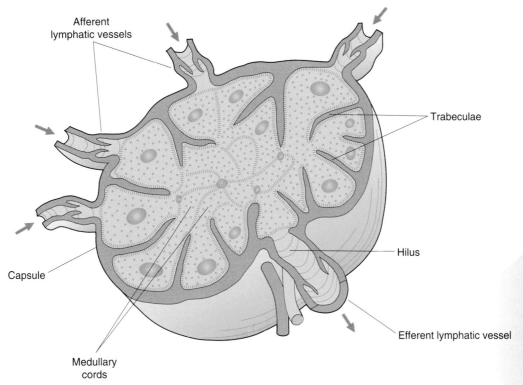

Afferent lymphatic vessels

Trabeculae

Hilus

Capsule

Efferent lymphatic vessel

Medullary cords

Figure 2.15   Cross-section of a lymphatic node.

of the swollen area. The volume of lymph passing into the capillaries and vessels depends on the pressure inside and outside the vessels.

Massage is very effective at speeding up the flow of lymph in the lymphatic vessels and thereby increasing the drainage of tissue fluid. Long effleurage strokes exert pressure and push the lymph along in the vessels towards the nearest set of lymphatic nodes (remember always move towards the nearest set of lymphatic nodes). The pressure (petrissage) manipulations squeeze the tissues. This pressure increases the amount of tissue fluid passing into the vessels to be drained away.

Functions of the lymphatic system

1   The lymphatic system drains tissue fluid from the spaces between cells.

2   It transports this tissue fluid and proteins to subclavian veins and so returns it back into the blood.

3   It transports fats from the small intestine to the blood.

| 4 | It produces lymphocytes, which protect and defend the body against infection and disease. |

| 5 | The nodes filter and remove broken-down foreign substances and waste. |

Effects of massage on the lymphatic system

◎ The flow of lymph in the lymphatic vessels is speeded up. As the hands move along in the direction of lymph drainage to the nearest group of lymphatic nodes, the speed of lymph flow is increased. Massage strokes should always be directed towards the nearest set of lymphatic nodes.

◎ Pressure on the tissues will facilitate the transfer of fluid across vessel walls. Fluid from the tissues will pass into the lymphatic vessels and will drain away more quickly; this will prevent or reduce oedema (swelling of the tissues).

◎ Larger particles of waste that are able to pass through the lymphatic vessel walls are removed more quickly.

The pressure and squeezing movements of petrissage are the most effective in reducing oedema, followed by effleurage. This effect is assisted if the part is elevated while being massaged, as gravity will assist drainage. Treatment of oedema using massage is described in Chapter 8.

❖ *The respiratory system* ❖

This system is responsible for the exchange of oxygen and carbon dioxide between the external environment and the internal environment of the body. It is closely linked with the cardio-vascular system, as the exchange of gases takes place between the alveoli of the lungs and the blood in the pulmonary capillaries.

The system is composed of the:

➤ nose and nasal passages

➤ pharynx

➤ larynx

➤ trachea

➤ bronchi and bronchioles

➤ lungs, which are composed of alveoli.

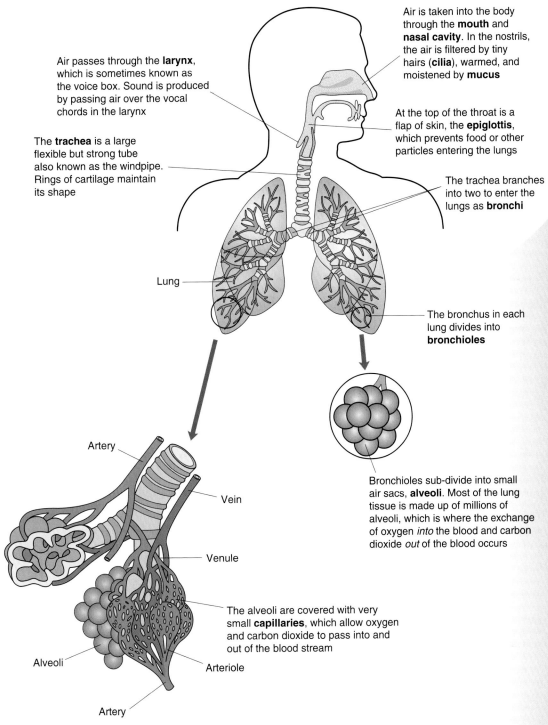

Air passes through the **larynx**, which is sometimes known as the voice box. Sound is produced by passing air over the vocal chords in the larynx

The **trachea** is a large flexible but strong tube also known as the windpipe. Rings of cartilage maintain its shape

Air is taken into the body through the **mouth** and **nasal cavity**. In the nostrils, the air is filtered by tiny hairs (**cilia**), warmed, and moistened by **mucus**

At the top of the throat is a flap of skin, the **epiglottis**, which prevents food or other particles entering the lungs

The trachea branches into two to enter the lungs as **bronchi**

Lung

The bronchus in each lung divides into **bronchioles**

Bronchioles sub-divide into small air sacs, **alveoli**. Most of the lung tissue is made up of millions of alveoli, which is where the exchange of oxygen *into* the blood and carbon dioxide *out* of the blood occurs

Artery

Vein

Venule

The alveoli are covered with very small **capillaries**, which allow oxygen and carbon dioxide to pass into and out of the blood stream

Alveoli

Arteriole

Artery

Figure 2.16   The respiratory system.

The nose

The nose serves as the first section of the passageway for air going into the lungs. It is also the organ of smell, as the olfactory receptors are located in the nose. The inner lining of the nose is a ciliated mucous membrane with a rich supply of blood vessels. It has two functions:

1 To filter the air as it enters the system, the tiny hairs trap organisms and dust particles, preventing their entry into the lungs.

2 To moisten and warm the air as it passes through.

The pharynx

Both the respiratory and digestive tracts share the pharynx, as both air and food pass through this passageway. The tonsils are located here.

The larynx

This is the voice box, which lies between the pharynx and the trachea. It is composed of cartilages and smooth muscle tissue. The larynx plays a part in respiration, speech and swallowing. Air passes through the larynx to the trachea: the passage of air over the vocal chords causes them to vibrate, producing sound. Between the base of the tongue and the upper opening of the larynx lies the *epiglottis*. This covers the larynx during the swallowing of food, protecting and shutting off the airway to prevent food entering.

The trachea

This is a tube about 11 centimetres long and 2.5 centimetres in diameter, which extends from the larynx to the bronchi. It is composed of smooth muscle with C-shaped bands of cartilage at regular intervals along its length. These cartilagenous bands prevent the walls of the trachea from collapsing inwards. The function of the trachea is to maintain a permanently open pathway to the lungs. Any obstruction of this vital airway, even for a few minutes, will result in asphyxia (suffocation) and death.

The bronchi

The trachea eventually divides into two primary bronchi:

- the right bronchus leads into the right lung
- the left bronchus leads into the left lung.

In structure, each bronchus is similar to the trachea, being composed of smooth muscle with C-shaped rings of cartilage at intervals along its length. As the bronchi enter the lungs they further subdivide into smaller secondary bronchi and then into even smaller bronchioles. The bronchioles further divide into minute tubes called alveolar ducts, which terminate in sponge-like sacs called alveoli.

The lungs

The left and right lungs are cone-shaped organs that extend from their base on the diaphragm below, to their apex above the clavicles. They lie within the thoracic cavity protected by the ribs and the sternum. The left lung is composed of two lobes and the right lung is composed of three lobes. They are covered by the visceral pleura containing serous fluid, which reduces friction and facilitates movement of the lungs during breathing. The lungs are composed of the tubes of the bronchial tree and the numerous sponge-like alveoli. The alveoli are surrounded by dense capillary networks. The function of the lungs is to provide a large surface area where the inspired air can come into close contact with the blood, thus facilitating the rapid exchange of gases. This exchange takes place across the alveoli–pulmonary capillary interface. Oxygen from inspired air diffuses through the walls of the alveoli, through the walls of the surrounding capillary networks, into the blood to be transported around the body to the tissue cells. Carbon dioxide from tissue cells is carried via the blood to the lungs. Here it diffuses through the capillary walls then through the walls of the alveoli to be expired out of the lungs. This gaseous exchange is regulated by the partial pressure of the gases in the alveolar air and in the pulmonary blood. The gases diffuse across the gradient from high pressure to low pressure until equilibrium is reached. (Diffusion is the movement of molecules across a permeable membrane.)

Ventilation

Ventilation is the movement of air in and out of the lungs. As explained previously, ventilation is brought about by the contraction of the skeletal muscles, which expands the thorax. The muscles involved are the diaphragm and the intercostal muscles that lie between the ribs. Ventilation is composed of *two* phases: *inspiration*, taking air into the lungs and *expiration*, expelling air out of the lungs.

During inspiration the external intercostal muscles contract, swinging the ribs outwards and upwards, rather like a bucket handle, and the sternum is pushed forward. This increases the thoracic cavity from side to side and from front to back. At the same time the diaphragm contracts to increase the cavity longitudinally. This increases the volume of the thorax and reduces the pressure within to below atmospheric pressure: consequently, air rushes into the lungs. During normal expiration these muscles relax, the thoracic cavity returns to its normal size, the pressure increases to above atmospheric pressure and air rushes out. During forced expiration the internal intercostals contract, pulling the ribs in and down: the diaphragm moves upwards, forcing air out.

Effects of massage on the respiratory system

The air passages are lined with a mucous membrane that continuously secretes a small quantity of mucus. This moistens the tubes and traps any organisms and particles in the inspired air. Any irritation of this membrane will result in an increase in the production of mucus. This mucus may thicken and become difficult to remove through coughing. Shaking and vibration manipulations performed over the chest can help to loosen these secretions so that they can be coughed up more easily. Deep breathing exercises will also help to move the mucus. See page 232.

❖ *The digestive system* ❖

The digestive system is concerned with the intake, breakdown and absorption of food substances. Carbohydrates, fats (lipids) and proteins are broken down into small molecules that can pass through the walls of the digestive tract into the bloodstream and then into body cells. Here they are used for energy, growth and repair of tissues.

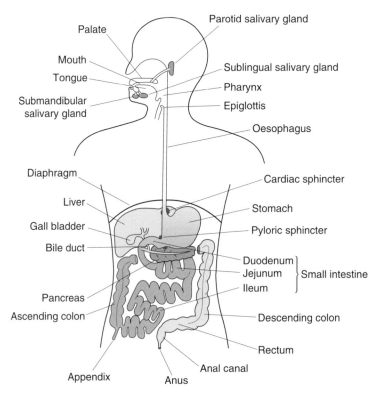

Figure 2.17   The digestive system.

The digestive system is divisible into two main parts:

1 **Gastro-intestinal tract** or alimentary canal: this is a tube approximately 7 m in length. It starts at the mouth and ends at the anus. The parts of the gastro-intestinal tract are:
- mouth
- pharynx
- oesophagus
- stomach
- small intestine, divided into duodenum, jejunum and ileum
- large intestine, divided into caecum, colon, rectum and anal canal.

2 **Accessory structures** and organs connect with the tract and play an important role in the digestive process. They are:
- teeth
- tongue
- salivary glands
- gall bladder
- pancreas
- liver.

Substances move along the tract by a series of muscle contractions known as **peristalsis**. Massage stimulates peristalsis and also aids the movement through the tract.

The digestive processes

The activities of the digestive system can be divided into four processes:

1 **Ingestion**: taking food into the body.

2 **Digestion**: the breaking down of food, which involves two processes:
- mechanical breakdown by chewing and movements of the tract that churns the food
- chemical breakdown by enzymes secreted into the tract at various stages, e.g. saliva from salivary glands in the mouth; gastric juices in the stomach; pancreatic juice from the pancreas; bile from the gall bladder; intestinal juice in the small intestine.

3 **Absorption**: the process by which digested food passes out of the tract into blood vessels and lymphatic capillaries and into cells.

4 **Elimination**: the passage of waste substances out of the body.

Digestion involves all the processes that break down and convert the food we eat into substances that can be absorbed and used by the body.

Food is broken down *mechanically* into minute particles and *chemically* into smaller molecules that are more easily absorbed. These changes begin as soon as food is taken into the mouth and continue through the gastro-intestinal tract until the processes of ingestion, digestion, absorption and elimination have been completed. The movement of food through the digestive system is by *peristalsis*: this is a wave-like contraction of the circular muscles in the wall of the intestines.

The mouth

Food is taken into the mouth, where the process of digestion begins. When the food is chewed the *teeth mechanically* break down food into small particles.

The salivary glands produce saliva, which pours into the mouth. This contains the enzyme AMYLASE (ptyalin), which begins the *chemical conversion* of starch into simple sugars. The food is moistened by the saliva and rolled by the tongue into a round ball called a *bolus.*

This is swallowed and passes through the pharynx into the oesophagus. It moves down the oesophagus by peristalsis into the stomach.

The stomach

This is a J-shaped sac that provides a reservoir for food and continues its breakdown. There are sphincters at the entrance and exit of the stomach that open and close to control the food coming in and passing out. Food can be held in the stomach for up to five hours while it is being digested.

The churning action of the stomach *mechanically* breaks the food down. The stomach produces gastric juices that break food down *chemically*.

The gastric juices include:

PEPSIN, which begins the chemical breakdown of protein to amino acids;
HYDROCHLORIC ACID, which aids digestion and destroys any ingested bacteria.

This mixture of partially digested food in the stomach is known as *chyme*. Very little *absorption* of food takes place in the stomach apart from water, alcohol and some drugs such as aspirin.

The small intestine

The small intestine is composed of three parts: duodenum, jejunum and ileum.

After the contents of the stomach are thoroughly churned, the chyme passes into the first part of the small intestine called the duodenum. In the duodenum, *bile* formed in the liver but stored in the gall bladder enters the tract to begin emulsifying (breaking down) fats into fatty acids.

Pancreatic juice from the pancreas also enters here, containing enzymes that further break down starches, proteins and fats.

➤ AMYLASE breaks down starch

➤ TRYPSIN breaks down proteins

➤ LIPASE emulsifies fats.

The juices from the mucous membrane lining the wall of the small intestine, containing LACTOSE, MALTOSE and SUCROSE, further break down sugars into GLUCOSE. The walls of the small intestine are lined with finger-like projections called VILLI that greatly increase the surface area, for *absorption* to take place. Each villus (singular) contains a network of blood and lymphatic capillaries. The digested, broken-down food products pass through the walls of the villi into the blood capillaries and hence into the bloodstream. Some fatty acids are absorbed into the lymphatic system and then returned in the lymph into the blood circulation via the thoracic duct.

The products that are not absorbed move on to the large intestine as waste.

The large intestine

This is divided into three parts: the *ascending colon*, which passes upwards on the right side of the abdomen; the *transverse colon*, which runs horizontally across the top of the abdomen and the *descending colon*, which passes downwards on the left side of the abdomen. This ends in the rectum and anus.

The colon reabsorbs water from the waste material as it passes through. Healthy bacteria in the colon also help to synthesise vitamins B and K. The colon forms the waste into faeces, which are stored in the rectum until they are *eliminated* through the anus.

Function of the parts of the gastro-intestinal tract

◎ **Mouth**
   ➤ Taking in of food (ingestion)
   ➤ Mechanical breakdown of food by chewing (mastication)
   ➤ Moistening and chemical breakdown of food by saliva
   ➤ The tongue rolls the food into a bolus for easy swallowing
   ➤ Swallowing moves food into the pharynx and the oesophagus.

◎ **Oesophagus**
   ➤ A tube through which food passes into the stomach. The food is moved along by the wave-like contraction and relaxation of the muscles surrounding the tract. This is known as peristalsis.

◎ **Stomach**
- ➤ Acts as a reservoir for food
- ➤ The mechanical breakdown of food continues by the churning motion of the stomach walls
- ➤ The chemical breakdown continues by the gastric juices
- ➤ Hydrochloric acid kills any bacteria in food
- ➤ Water, certain drugs and alcohol are absorbed through the walls into the bloodstream.

◎ **Small intestine**
- ➤ Controls the secretion of bile and pancreatic juice, which further break down food
- ➤ Intestinal juices complete the *digestion* of food
- ➤ *Absorption* of the digested food through the walls of the villi and into the blood; fat passes into the lymph
- ➤ Waste is passed on to the large intestine.

◎ **Large intestine**
- ➤ Absorbs water from the waste matter and returns it to the blood
- ➤ Good bacteria in the gut form vitamins B and K
- ➤ Stores and forms waste into faeces
- ➤ *Eliminates* waste in the form of faeces through the rectum and anus.

Effects of massage on the digestive system

◎ Abdominal massage stimulates peristalsis and the movement of digested food through the colon.

◎ Massage may be helpful to relieve constipation and flatulence.

❖ *The nervous system* ❖

The nervous system is the communication and control system of the body. It works with the endocrine system to maintain homeostasis (body balance). The nervous system will sense changes inside and outside the body, interpret them and initiate appropriate action. The nervous system is made up of the:

- ➤ **central** nervous system, comprising the brain and spinal cord

- ➤ **peripheral** nervous system, comprising 12 pairs of cranial nerves arising from the brain and 31 pairs of spinal nerves arising from the spinal cord

- ➤ **autonomic** system.

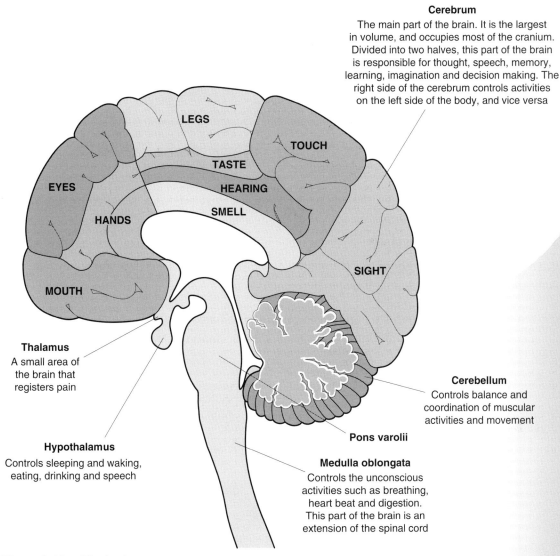

Cerebrum
The main part of the brain. It is the largest in volume, and occupies most of the cranium. Divided into two halves, this part of the brain is responsible for thought, speech, memory, learning, imagination and decision making. The right side of the cerebrum controls activities on the left side of the body, and vice versa

LEGS
TOUCH
TASTE
HEARING
SMELL
EYES
HANDS
SIGHT
MOUTH

Thalamus
A small area of the brain that registers pain

Cerebellum
Controls balance and coordination of muscular activities and movement

Pons varolii

Hypothalamus
Controls sleeping and waking, eating, drinking and speech

Medulla oblongata
Controls the unconscious activities such as breathing, heart beat and digestion. This part of the brain is an extension of the spinal cord

Figure 2.18   The brain.

The peripheral nerves carry impulses inwards from sensory receptors in sense organs to the brain. They also carry impulses from the brain to muscles and glands.

Nervous tissue is composed of functional units called *neurones*, which conduct impulses, and the supporting tissue called *neuroglia*.

There are three types of neurone:

1 **Sensory** neurones, which transmit stimuli *from* sensory organs *to* the spinal cord and brain. They convey sensations of pain, pressure, temperature, taste, sight etc.

2 **Motor** neurones, which transmit stimuli *from* the brain and spinal cord *to* muscles and glands. They initiate the contraction of muscles and the action of glands.

3 **Interneurons**, which form connections between neurones. They convey impulses from one neurone to another.

Structure of a neurone

All neurones have a similar structure: they have a **cell body**, one long nerve fibre called an **axon** and several short nerve fibres called **dendrites**.

Axons carry impulses *away* from the cell body; dendrites carry impulses *towards* the cell body.

The nerve impulse

When receptors or sense organs are stimulated, an impulse is initiated that is transmitted along the sensory nerve towards the spinal cord and brain.

The brain then decides upon the corrective action and initiates impulses that are transmitted along the motor nerves to appropriate muscles or glands. Impulses are transmitted in axons

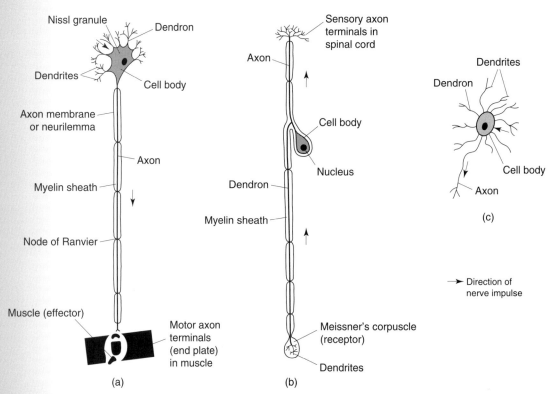

Figure 2.19 Types of neurone: (a) motor neurone (b) sensory neurone (c) inter neurone.

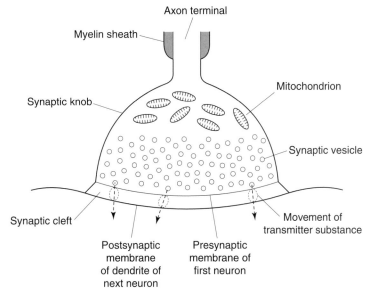

Figure 2.20   Conduction of nerve impulse across synapse.

and dendrites in one direction only as shown in Figure 2.20. More than one neuron will be involved in the transmission of a nerve impulse and the point at which the impulse passes from one neuron to another is called a synapse.

Synapse
Nerve-to-nerve junction

A synapse is the point where two neurones connect. The neurones do not make direct contact: there is a gap between them called a *synaptic cleft*. The nerve impulse must be transmitted across this gap. Chemicals called neurotransmitters conduct the impulses across the gap: these chemicals may facilitate the passage of the impulse or they may inhibit the passage of the impulse:

- acetylcholine (Ach) facilitates the passage of an impulse
- gamma-aminobutyric acid (GABA) inhibits the passage of an impulse.

Nerve-to-muscle junction

The point at which a nerve connects with its muscle fibre is known as the *neuro-muscular junction*, which is very similar to a synapse. The impulse is transmitted across the gap from the axon end of the nerve to the *motor end plate* on the muscle fibre, by the chemical transmitter acetylcholine.

Receptors

The nervous system has millions of receptors, which are the distal ends of the dendrites of the sensory nerves. These receptors detect changes in the external and internal environment. All sensations are felt through the stimulation of these receptors. In response to these stimuli, nerve impulses are initiated and transmitted along the nerve to the spinal cord and brain, where they are interpreted and the appropriate responses selected. For example, if the receptors register cold, these stimuli are conducted to the brain. Here they are interpreted and the brain sends impulses to stimulate muscles to contract rapidly: this produces body heat, which we know as shivering.

The main groups of receptors are:

Exteroceptors: there are many types, which tend to lie on the surface of the body: they detect changes in the external environment. They are found in skin, mucous membranes, and register cold, heat, touch, pressure, pain etc. Highly specialised ones are found in the eye and ear for sight and sound. Those in the skin include Meissner's corpuscles, which sense light touch, Merkel's discs sense touch and stretch, and Pacinian corpuscles sense deep pressure.

Interoceptors or visceroceptors: these lie internally and detect changes in the internal environment. They are found in the internal organs such as the intestine, stomach, liver, kidneys etc and in the walls of blood vessels. These register changes in the internal organs.

Proprioceptors: these are located in muscles, tendons and joints and register the degree of stretch or tension in a muscle while others provide information of joint position and the spatial location of body parts.

Reflexes

There are many types of physiological reflex resulting in responses, such as coughing, sneezing, blinking: these are involuntary actions, and are not under conscious control.

Reflex action

A reflex action is a rapid involuntary response to a stimulus. When a rapid response to a particular stimulus is required the impulses do not always ascend to the brain, they simply enter the spinal cord, where an automatic response is initiated.

A reflex arc

This is the pathway taken by an impulse, from the sensory receptors in the skin, along the sensory nerve into the spinal cord, via an interneuron and along the motor nerve to the muscles, which contract in response.

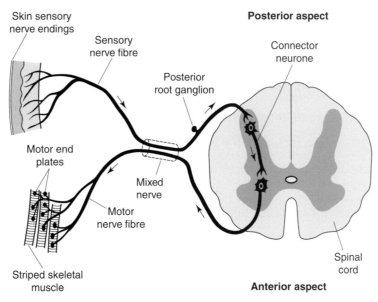

Figure 2.21   A simple three-neurone reflex arc.

EXAMPLE

If a hot object is touched, the sensory nerve endings in the skin register something hot and the flexor muscles of the arm will contract to withdraw the hand.

Pain

Palpation or massage of the tissues may produce pain. The pain may be in the exact location of the problem and may be due to increased tension in the underlying tissues or the pain may be referred from another area. Problems affecting internal organs may refer tension and pain to an area of skin and subcutaneous tissue whose sensory fibres share the same spinal segment as the nerve supply of the affected organ. Specific neuromuscular techniques over that area will produce an automatic reflex response in the affected organ. Tension points or nodules that become chronic can develop into trigger points. These may lie deep within a muscle but may refer pain to another area called the target zone, which shares the same nerve pathway.

The autonomic system

The autonomic system consists of two parts: the sympathetic and the parasympathetic parts, which exercise involuntary control of smooth muscle, cardiac muscle, and glands. The sympathetic system has similar effects on the body as those produced by the hormones adrenaline and noradrenaline: they bring about physiological changes that help the body to cope quickly under conditions of stress, the fight and flight reaction. Stimulation of the sympathetic system tends to speed up processes while stimulation of the parasympathetic system tends to slow things down. The systems work together to maintain a stable internal environment.

Stimulation of *the sympathetic system* causes the following changes:

- the heart rate and strength of contraction increases
- the coronary arteries dilate, increasing the blood supply to the heart
- contraction of the spleen increases the volume of circulating blood
- the blood supply to the organs of digestion decreases thus providing more blood for skeletal muscle contraction
- the rate of respiration, oxygen consumption and carbon dioxide output increases
- increase in the rate of conversion of glycogen, making more glucose available for energy
- increase in the quantity of sweat secreted, with increased heat loss
- the pupils dilate giving a wide-eyed look

Stimulation of *the parasympathetic system* balances the effect of the sympathetic system, producing opposite effects:

- slows the heart rate and decreases the strength of contraction
- constricts coronary arteries, decreasing the blood supply to the heart
- reduces the rate of respiration and oxygen consumption
- increases blood supply to the digestive system and stimulates peristalsis
- constricts the pupils.

During massage the sensory receptors in the skin convey impulses of touch and pressure to the central nervous system. If pressure is too light it can be irritating; if it is too deep or uneven it may be irritating or painful. Muscles then respond with increased tension. Slow, rhythmical, deep massage has a soothing effect on the nerve endings, promoting relaxation.

Effects of massage on the nervous system

- ◎ Slow, rhythmical massage produces a soothing, sedative effect on sensory nerve endings, promoting general relaxation.

- ◎ Vigorous brisk massage will have a stimulating effect, producing feelings of vigour and glow. Light hacking on either side of the vertebral column is particularly effective.

- ◎ If massage technique is poor or too heavy, the pain sensors in the skin will be stimulated. Painful manipulations will increase tension, which is counter-productive, and care must be taken to avoid this. Similarly, if movements are too light, i.e. barely touching the skin or tickling, this will have an irritating effect that will also increase tension and must be avoided.

❖ *The urinary system* ❖

The urinary system is *one* of the excretory systems of the body.

The body takes in food, liquid and air, all of which are necessary for the metabolic activities of cells that sustain life. These metabolic processes release waste substances that must be eliminated from the body.

Excretory organs

◎ The *excretory organs* of the body are the kidneys, skin, lungs and large intestine.

◎ The kidneys form urine, which passes to the bladder and is excreted through urination.

◎ The skin eliminates water and mineral salts through perspiration.

◎ The large intestine eliminates waste from digested food through defecation.

◎ The lungs eliminate carbon dioxide and water vapour through exhalation.

The urinary system is made up of:

➤ two kidneys – which filter the blood and form urine

➤ two ureters – two tubes that carry urine from the kidneys to the bladder

➤ the bladder – a hollow sac where urine is stored until it is excreted

➤ the urethra – a tube that carries the urine from the bladder out of the body.

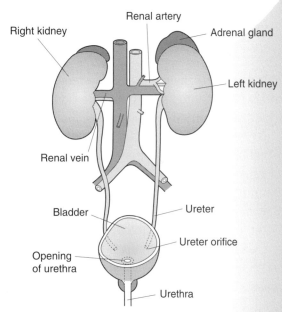

Figure 2.22   The urinary system. Top of bladder removed to show openings.

The kidneys

The kidneys are bean-shaped organs approximately 10 cm in length. They are situated on the posterior wall of the abdominal cavity and lie on either side of the spine at the level between the twelfth thoracic and the third lumbar vertebrae. Their medial surface is concave and has an indentation or notch called the *hilum*. They are covered and held in place by fibrous connective tissue and protected by adipose tissue (fat), which insulates and protects the kidneys.

Blood is brought to the kidneys via the renal artery and taken away via the renal vein. These vessels enter the kidney at the hilum, together with the nerves and lymphatic vessels. One ureter leaves each kidney at the hilum and leads into the bladder.

The kidneys are composed of three distinct layers:

1 a tough fibrous outer layer or capsule that encases and protects the kidney

2 the cortex, which lies in the middle, and is dark red in colour

3 the medulla, which is the inner layer, and is reddish brown in colour.

Each kidney is made up of over a million functional units called **nephrons**, where the kidney processes of *filtration* and *selective reabsorption* occur (Figure 2.24).

Blood entering the kidney via the renal artery passes into fine capillary networks, which surround the tubules of the nephrons. The first phase of kidney function is the *filtration* of substances from the capillary blood into the kidney. These substances pass from the blood in the glomerulus into the Bowman's capsule of the kidney: they include water, mineral salts, glucose, toxins, uric acid and urea. These pass through the tubules to be eliminated but some substances are reabsorbed if the body needs them.

The substances to be eliminated from the body form urine and include the waste products of protein metabolism, i.e. urea, uric acid, ammonia; toxins; certain mineral salts and some water. These substances pass along the tubules into the ureters and bladder to be eliminated.

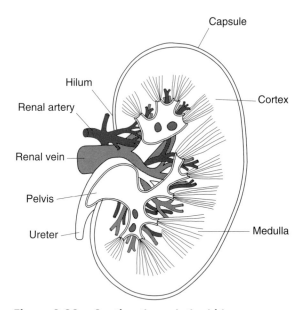

Figure 2.23   Section through the kidney.

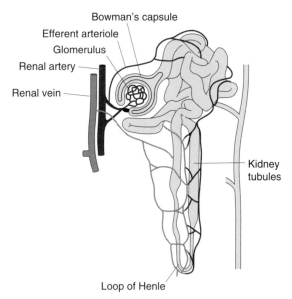

Figure 2.24   The nephron.

Other substances, needed by the body, are reabsorbed into the bloodstream. These substances pass from the kidney tubules back into the capillary blood: this is known as *selective reabsorption*. Most of the water, all of the glucose, some sodium ions and vitamin C are reabsorbed into the blood. Hormones regulate the reabsorption of water and sodium depending on body requirements.

Through these functions of filtration and reabsorption, the kidneys adjust the balance of water, sodium ions and other substances leaving the body, with those entering the body. In this way the kidneys regulate the composition and volume of blood and maintain a stable internal environment for the tissues, known as homeostasis.

Functions of the kidney:

◎ formation of urine

◎ elimination of toxic waste substances that are harmful to the body

◎ regulation of water balance in the body

◎ regulation of sodium level and other electrolytes

◎ maintenance of normal pH level of the blood

◎ the kidneys also influence blood pressure.

These functions of the kidneys maintain homeostasis and are vital for sustaining life: kidney failure will result in death. Kidney dialysis is a treatment for maintaining life if the kidneys fail to function. The patient is connected to a machine that circulates their blood through special tubing immersed in dialysing fluid containing prescribed substances necessary for treatment. Any unwanted or harmful substances are removed from the blood and its constituents are balanced. The procedure must be carried out at regular intervals to sustain life. A kidney transplant will offer the chance of near normal life to those fortunate enough to receive one. Unfortunately, there are not enough kidneys available to meet the demand.

The ureters

The right and left ureters are two tubes extending from the kidneys to the bladder. The upper end opens out into a funnel called the renal pelvis where the urine is collected. The ureter leaves the hilum of the kidney, and its lower end enters the posterior surface of the bladder. There is a small valve at this entrance to the bladder that shuts to prevent the backward flow of urine when the bladder is full.

The walls of the ureters are composed of three coats: an inner lining of mucous membrane, a middle coat made of two layers of smooth muscle, and an outer fibrous coat. Urine is collected from the kidney and moved along the ureters by peristalsis (wave-like contractions of the muscle wall) to the bladder.

The bladder

The bladder is a muscular sac that acts as a reservoir for the urine. Its walls are composed of three layers of smooth muscle lined with a mucous membrane. The bladder is capable of distension, which occurs as the bladder fills. Stretch receptors in the bladder wall stimulate an awareness that the bladder needs to be emptied and also initiate a reflex contraction of the bladder. At the same time there is a reflex relaxation of the internal sphincter followed by relaxation of the external sphincter, and the bladder empties. The passage of urine through the urethra, known as micturition, occurs when the two sphincters controlling the opening relax.

It is possible to control the passage of urine out of the urethra by voluntary contraction of the external sphincter. The ability to exercise this control will diminish if there is nerve damage, or the sphincter muscle is weak: voluntary control is lost and urine leaks out of the urethra. The leakage is worse if abdominal pressure is increased as in coughing or laughing. This involuntary passage of urine is known as urinary incontinence. Many women suffer from this condition especially after childbirth when the pelvic floor muscles are stretched, or with ageing when the muscles lose tone. This condition can be helped and these women should be encouraged to seek medical advice.

Effects of massage on the urinary system

Massage movements, and in particular abdominal massage, will improve the circulation to the kidney and may slightly increase the output of urine and hence the elimination of toxins.

Precautions

Heavy percussion manipulations should not be performed over the area of the kidneys as there is a risk of damage.

When massaging the abdomen, too heavy a pressure over the bladder area can be uncomfortable.

Pain in the lower thoracic and lumbar region radiating around to the abdomen on one side may indicate a kidney problem. If you are unsure of the cause of pain in this loin region, seek medical advice.

Make sure that the client empties the bladder before treatment, as it is impossible to relax if the bladder is full.

❖ *The endocrine system* ❖

The endocrine system is made up of separate glands located in different parts of the body. Each gland makes chemical substances called hormones, which regulate and influence body processes such as growth, development, metabolism, reproduction and responses to stress.

The endocrine system and the nervous system control and co-ordinate body functions and maintain the body's internal balanced state (homeostasis).

Endocrine glands are known as ductless glands because the hormones they secrete pour directly into the bloodstream (unlike exocrine glands, which pass their secretions into ducts, e.g. sebaceous glands).

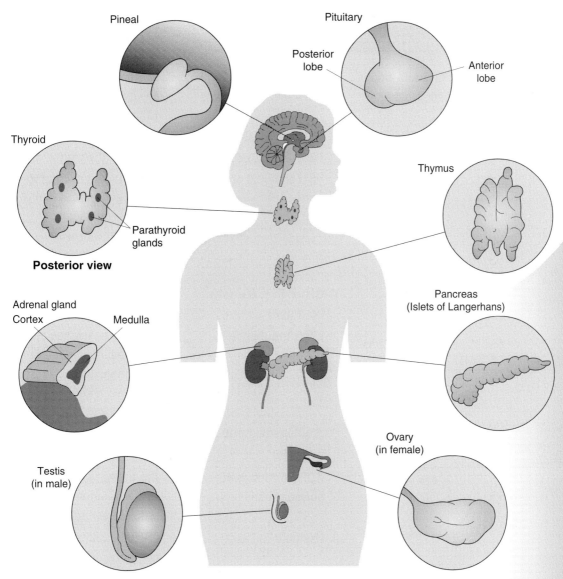

Figure 2.25 The endocrine system.

Hormones are known as chemical messengers. They are released from the gland and carried by the bloodstream to their target organs. One gland may produce a number of different hormones that influence and control the activities of many organs. The responses in the target organ are usually slow and continue over a long period of time. Some endocrine glands control the function of other endocrine glands.

The *pituitary gland* controls the function of other glands and because of this it is known as the 'Master Gland'.

Table 2.3 Classification of endocrine glands

Gland	Location	Hormone	Function
Pituitary (Anterior)	Cranium under the brain	ACTH (Adrinocorticotropin)	Promotes development of the adrenal cortex; helps in conditions of stress
		TSH (Thyroid-stimulating hormone) thyrotropin	Stimulates the thyroid to produce thyroxin
		FSH (Follicle-stimulating hormone)	Stimulates growth and oestrogen production of ovarian follicles; stimulates growth of testes; promotes the development of sperm
		GH or STH (Growth hormone)	Promotes growth of all body tissues
		LH (Luteinising hormone)	Stimulates ovaries and the production of oestrogen and progesterone in females; stimulates testosterone in males
		(Lactogenic hormone) prolactin	Stimulates secretion of milk by the breasts
Pituitary (Posterior)	Base of the brain	ADH (Antidiuretic hormone)	Promotes reabsorption of water in kidney tubules; reduces volume of urine
		Oxytocin	Causes contraction of pregnant uterus. Stimulates flow of milk from breasts
Adrenal cortex	Above the upper end of the kidney	Cortisol	Aids in metabolism; active to reduce stress
		Aldosterone	Helps to regulate sodium and potassium levels in the blood
		(Sex hormones)	Contribute to the secondary sexual characteristics in males

(continued)

Table 2.3 (*continued*)

Gland	Location	Hormone	Function
Adrenal medulla	Above the upper end of each kidney	Androgens Adrenaline	Stimulates smooth and cardiac muscle; increases BMR, blood pressure and heart rate; prepares for fight and flight
Pancreas (Islets of Langerhans)	Below the stomach	Insulin	Helps the transport of glucose into cells; decreases blood sugar levels
		Glucagon	Increases blood sugar levels
Parathyroid	In the throat in front of the trachea	Parathyrin	Increases calcium level in blood
Thyroid	In the throat in front of the trachea	Thyroxin	Regulates metabolic rate, growth and development of tissues
		Calcitonin	Decreases calcium level in blood
Ovaries (Ovarian)	Each side of the uterus	Oestrogens	Stimulates the growth of sexual follicle organs, e.g. uterus, breasts etc
Corpus luteum	In the ovaries	Progesterone	Stimulates the development of the breasts. Helps in maintaining pregnancy
Testes	In the scrotum	Testosterone	Stimulates development of sexual organs. Stimulates hair growth on the body and face
Thymus	Behind the sternum	Thymosin	Stimulates the production of antibodies by lymphocytes
Pineal	In the brain	Melatonin	Inhibits LH secretion and affects body rhythms

Under normal conditions the amount of hormone produced and secreted by the glands is carefully regulated by the nervous system. Under- or over-production of a hormone can result in a number of endocrine disorders.

❖ *Psychological effects of massage* ❖

The psychological effects of massage must also be considered.

→ It creates feelings of well-being and health.

→ It promotes feelings of vigour and increases energy.

→ It increases postural awareness.

→ It promotes feelings of being cared for and cosseted, which in turn promote relaxation, contentment and satisfaction.

→ It reduces mental stress, which also enhances feelings of contentment and relaxation.

QUESTIONS

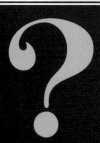

1. Give the organisational levels of the body.
2. Explain briefly the structure of a typical cell.
3. Name the largest of the organelles and explain its importance.
4. List the three types of cartilage and state where each type is found.
5. Briefly outline the structure of the skin.
6. Explain any four functions of the skin.
7. Describe four ways in which massage will improve the condition of the skin.
8. Explain how you would adapt a body massage for the older client with dry, thin, wrinkled skin.
9. List the bones that form:
   (a) The axial skeleton
   (b) The appendicular skeleton
10. Draw and label a diagram of a synovial joint.
11. Explain four functions of the skeleton.
12. Give three beneficial effects resulting from massage performed around a joint.
13. List the three types of muscle tissue and state where each is found.
14. Name the muscle tissue that forms the body flesh and produces body movement.
15. Briefly explain how massage will increase the blood supply to a muscle.
16. Explain four effects of massage on muscle tissue.
17. Give the function of the cardio-vascular system.
18. Name the four chambers of the heart.
19. Give three differences between the blood transported in arteries and the blood transported in veins.
20. Massage produces 'hyperaemia' and 'erythema'. Explain what is meant by these terms.
21. List and explain the component parts of the lymphatic system.
22. Name two groups of lymphatic nodes found in the leg and two groups of lymphatic nodes found in the arm.
23. Give four functions of the lymphatic system.
24. Give four effects of massage on the lymphatic system.
25. Briefly explain the four functions of the digestive system.
26. List the parts of the gastro-intestinal tract.
27. Name four accessory organs of digestion.

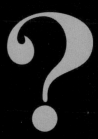

28. Name and explain the process by which food moves along the digestive tract.
29. Give the function of the respiratory system.
30. List the component parts of the respiratory system.
31. Explain what is meant by:
    (a) inspiration
    (b) expiration
32. Describe the mechanism of inspiration and expiration.
33. Give the function of the nervous system.
34. Name the three main parts of the nervous system.
35. Select one correct answer to the following statement:
    All sensation is felt through the stimulation of ...
    (a) motor end plate
    (b) receptors
    (c) neuroglia
36. Define the following:
    (a) reflex arc
    (b) reflex action
37. Give the function of the urinary system.
38. List the parts that make up the urinary system.
39. Name the two processes that take place in the nephrons.
40. List the five functions of the kidney.
41. Which of the following statements is correct?
    (a) hormones produce effects quickly
    (b) hormones produce effects slowly.
42. Name the endocrine glands and give their location.
43. Name one hormone that increases blood sugar levels.
44. Name the gland known as the master gland and state why it is so called.

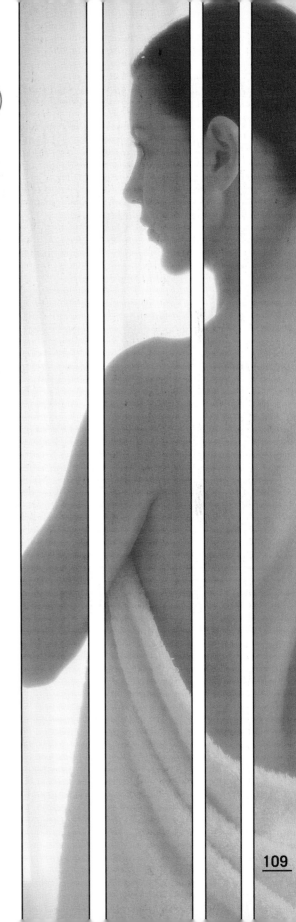

Part B

Consultation, preparation and massage movements

3 Professional conduct, ethics and preparation

OBJECTIVES

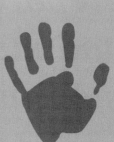

After you have studied this chapter you will be able to:
1. explain what is meant by the term 'ethics'
2. list the factors that contribute to professional behaviour
3. explain why safety and hygiene are important to the therapist
4. discuss the factors to consider when preparing the working area
5. prepare the working area
6. discuss the important factors to consider when selecting a massage couch
7. prepare a massage couch for treatment
8. discuss the procedure for preparing the working trolley
9. prepare the working trolley
10. explain the importance of having a selection of massage lubricants on the trolley
11. give the factors that contribute to high standards of personal hygiene
12. discuss the psychological preparation for massage
13. explain how you would prepare and position a client for massage
14. prepare and position a client for massage
15. discuss the importance and purpose of detailed consultation
16. carry out a detailed consultation
17. recognise the importance of keeping accurate records of every procedure
18. list the essential information required on a record card
19. design a record card for use in massage
20. list the contra-indications to massage
21. recognise the conditions where medical advice must be sought
22. identify conditions where extra care must be taken
23. recognise the importance of explaining and agreeing the treatment plan with the client including the purpose, long-term objective, time scale and cost.

❖ *Ethics* ❖

Ethics refers to the standards and conduct of behaviour of an individual or professional group. Massage therapists must undergo a course of reputable training to enable them to acquire the understanding and skills necessary to carry out safe and effective treatment. In addition, they must consider their standard of behaviour in relation to colleagues, clients and the general public.

A high standard of professional conduct will gain the confidence of clients and establish an excellent reputation, which is the basis for success. Abide by the following code of practices:

1   Look professional – be clean, neat and tidy.

2   Be punctual, keep appointments, do not cancel at the last minute. Always be on time for work.

3   Be discreet and refrain from gossip. Remember that clients often confide personal problems during consultation. These facts and all personal details must be treated with the utmost confidentiality. Do not repeat information or gossip to colleagues or others.

4   Be loyal to your employer and colleagues; create a friendly working relationship with all.

5   Be honest and reliable – this will gain the trust of others and establish a high reputation. Do not make false claims for treatments, but explain the benefits fairly. Be honest when advertising.

6   Speak correctly and politely to everyone. Do not use improper language. Consider the manner in which you answer or speak on the telephone. Be competent, helpful and pleasant.

7   Be polite and courteous at all times. There will be difficult clients to deal with – learn to handle tricky situations with tact and diplomacy.

8   Know and abide by legal requirements and local authority bye-laws, rules and regulations for conducting your business.

9   Keep up to date with new theories, techniques and treatments. Attend courses on a regular basis and keep in touch with other professionals in your field.

10   Always practise the highest standards of personal and salon hygiene.

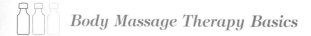

11 Do your utmost to deliver the most effective treatment suited to the needs of the client.

12 Organise yourself and your business to ensure a smooth-running, efficient service for the benefit of all concerned.

❖ *Client consultation* ❖

Initial consultation

The consultation is a very important part of the treatment – sufficient time must be allowed so that it is not rushed. This is the time to gather and exchange information.

The initial consultation will be the longest and provide detailed information, which must be accurately recorded on a treatment card. This must be filed in a safe and accessible place and used each time the client attends for treatment. Before subsequent treatments, a brief consultation is usually sufficient to establish the effects and outcomes of the previous treatments and whether any changes are to be made or further action is to be taken.

For the consultation the client should be seated comfortably, with the therapist positioned alongside or opposite. The environment should feel warm and private.

Detailed consultation is important for the following reasons:

◎ to introduce yourself and get to know the client

◎ to establish a rapport with the client and put her/him at ease

◎ to develop mutual trust and gain the client's confidence

◎ to gain information on the client's past and present state of mental and physical health

◎ to identify any contra-indications

◎ to gain insight into the client's lifestyle, responsibilities, work environment, leisure activities etc

◎ to identify the client's needs and expectations of the treatment

◎ to establish the most appropriate form of treatment and to discuss and agree this with the client

◎ to explain the treatment fully to the client, including the procedure, expected effects, timing and frequency

◎ to agree a treatment plan, the timing and cost with the client so that s/he fully understands the financial commitment, and obtain a signed consent form

◎ to answer queries and questions related to the treatment and to allay doubts and fears.

The information gathered will provide a baseline from which the appropriate treatment is planned, the effectiveness of the treatment can be judged and any necessary changes or adjustments made.

Note: all the information given must be recorded and treated in confidence.

Essential information

The following personal, medical and environmental factors should be recorded on the consultation card:

PERSONAL DETAILS

◎ status

◎ name

◎ address

◎ date of birth

◎ home and work telephone numbers

◎ occupation

◎ doctor's name, address and telephone number

These details will enable you to contact the client quickly should you need to cancel or change an appointment or for any other reason. They will also enable you to seek advice from his/her doctor should this be necessary.

PAST MEDICAL HISTORY

◎ surgical operations

◎ pregnancies

◎ serious illness

These details will enable you to establish the client's state of health; the likelihood of any contra-indications as a result of past illnesses; whether particular care must be taken over certain areas and whether medical referral is necessary. If the client suffers from a condition that is an absolute contra-indication (see page 115 on), then massage must not be given.

PRESENT MEDICAL HISTORY

◎ medication

◎ general health

◎ current treatments

◎ identification of stress: work, home or other sources

These details will indicate whether massage will be helpful to this client and will influence the type of massage to be given, e.g. if the client is stressed then a relaxing massage will be the choice. If there is pain and stiffness then the massage will be adapted to meet these needs.

MASSAGE ANALYSIS

◎ contra-indications

◎ has client received massage in the past?

◎ how long ago?

◎ number of sessions

◎ did client benefit from the massage?

◎ reasons for requesting massage

These details will again highlight contra-indications that will indicate whether massage would be suitable for the client. They will also provide information regarding the client's previous experience of massage. Did s/he find it beneficial, are there any preferences, likes and dislikes that should be recorded?

EXAMINATION

◎ posture

◎ height

◎ weight

SKIN CONDITIONS

◎ skin type: smooth/supple; dry/flaky; loose/stretched

◎ stretch marks

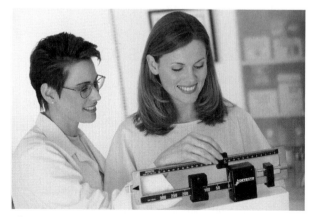

Figure 3.1   Initial client consultation.

◎ areas of hard fat/cellulite

◎ areas of soft fat

◎ general muscle tone

◎ bony protuberances

◎ fluid retention

◎ disfiguration or distortion of surface anatomy

◎ other factors that may affect massage

These details will enable you to select the appropriate massage and massage medium to be used for the client, e.g. clients with dry flaky skin will require a suitably lubricating medium; thin crêpy skin and bony protuberances will require lighter manipulations. They will also indicate the depth and adaptations necessary to suit the client, e.g. hard fat can take more pressure than soft fat, but areas of cellulite can be painful if pressure is too great. Well-toned clients often prefer a brisker, deeper massage than clients with poor muscle tone. Details of posture, height and weight must be recorded at the beginning of the treatment and compared throughout the course.

OTHER INFORMATION

◎ reasons for requesting massage

◎ expectations from the treatment

◎ any concerns or worries

This information will help you to formulate the best treatment plan to meet the needs of the client. The plan should then be fully explained to the client; s/he must be given the opportunity to ask questions and given full answers to allay any concerns or fears. The long-term objective, the cost and timing must be agreed and a consent form signed by the client.

❖ *Contra-indications to massage* ❖

Understanding contra-indications

Massage must always be given to bring about improvement, either of specific conditions, or the general well-being of each client. Clients should always feel that the treatment is beneficial and helping them to achieve their desired results. Massage should never be given if there is any risk of harming the client or making any condition worse.

Every therapist has a legal responsibility under the health, safety and welfare legislation to protect him/herself and the clients from harm. Remember that if the client is harmed in any way s/he may make a claim against you. You must therefore ensure that you have not been negligent in any way, that you have selected the appropriate treatment and that you have a written record of the consultation, the treatment given and the aftercare advice.

During the consultation you must decide whether massage is appropriate, safe and suitable for the client. If the client is suffering from any condition that could be aggravated or made worse by massage then obviously the treatment must not be carried out. These conditions are known as 'contra-indications' to massage. Knowledge of the potential harmful effects of inappropriate massage is extremely important and so is the ability to recognise contra-indications.

The effects of massage may be harmful in certain circumstances. The following explanations will help you to understand why massage should not be carried out if certain conditions are present. There are dangers associated with the following:

1. Cardio-vascular problems

Massage is thought to increase blood flow, which is desirable in many conditions, but can be dangerous in others. Infection and cancer cells can be carried around the body in the bloodstream to affect other areas. Bruised, damaged or broken blood vessels would be further damaged by massage, resulting in increased bleeding. Varicose veins should be avoided as the tissues around the vein may be fragile and easily damaged and there is a tendency for the stagnating blood to form clots. Massage proximal to the vein may prevent these problems.

The greatest danger occurs if the client suffers from phlebitis or thrombosis, or both, known as thrombophlebitis. When a vein in the calf becomes inflamed (phlebitis), massage may increase the inflammation but the greatest danger is if a clot develops in the vein (thrombosis). When the circulation of blood slows down, platelets and fibrin adhere to the blood vessel wall, forming a clot. While it is attached it is called a *thrombus*.

The clot or a portion of it may become dislodged, and float in the blood: it is then called an *embolus*. This will move through the bloodstream and may cause a blockage in a smaller vein. If this happens in the lungs it could be fatal.

Dislodging or fragmenting a blood clot is the greatest danger of massage as it could result in death if medical treatment is not administered quickly.

Thrombosis usually develops in the calf or hamstrings. Be alert and suspect this condition if a client complains of deep pain in the calf or back of thigh. There may be swelling of the area and the muscles may feel tense and hard. Refer to a doctor or hospital immediately.

2. Lymphatic drainage

The lymphatic system removes excess fluid from all over the body, returning it into the bloodstream. Lymph transports the larger particles of waste from the tissues as well as bacteria, viruses or cancerous substances. Because massage increases lymphatic flow, the rate at which these toxic substances are carried and spread around the body is increased. Be particularly aware if the client has swollen or painful lymph glands; do not massage, and seek medical advice.

3. Skin contact and friction

As the hands move over the client's skin, any bacterial, viral or fungal infections can be spread over the skin to a non-infected area or onto the therapist's hands. Infections may be transmitted from client to therapist or from therapist to client in this way.

Friction of the hands may open healing wounds or abrasions. This will expose the area to infection by micro-organisms. There will also be a risk of blood contamination between the client and the therapist. Blood contamination must be avoided, as serious life-threatening viruses and diseases such as Hepititis B and HIV (AIDS) can be transmitted in this way.

(Remember that infection may pass from client to client via the commodities such as pillows, towels, sheets etc. Infestation by parasites such as lice, fleas and itch mites can be passed in the same way.)

4. The healing process

Any injury or damage to the tissues or fractures of bones must be allowed to heal completely before massage is given to the area. If massage is given before healing is complete, there is a danger of further damage to the tissues and delaying the healing process.

5. Pins and plates

If massage is performed over an area where pins and plates have been inserted to stabilise bones and joints, there is a danger of their becoming loose, and also, through the pressure of massage over any protruding parts, there is a danger of damaging the surrounding soft tissues.

6. Allergic reactions

The oil or cream etc. used as the massage medium may cause an allergic reaction in some clients. This will produce an excessive erythema: the area becoming very red and hot or a rash may appear. Remove the medium immediately and wash in warm water.

7. Fragile skin

There is always a danger of breaking down fragile, thin skin, causing open wounds. Particular care must be taken with diabetics and anyone on steroid treatments as the skin may be fragile and healing may be slow. Plenty of lubrication and light pressure only must be used.

Conditions where massage is contra-indicated

A contra-indication is a condition that, if present, means that the treatment should not be carried out.

Some conditions mean that massage is totally contra-indicated and must not be performed to any part of the body. These are known as *absolute contra-indications*.

Other conditions prevent massage over the local area of the condition, but other non-affected areas or limbs may be massaged: these are known as *local contra-indications*.

Absolute contra-indications to massage

Do not massage if the following contra-indications are present:

◎ Cancer: any client with cancer or a history of cancer must not be massaged, as cancer cells may be spread through the lymphatic system. If you are unsure, seek medical advice. Be particularly aware if a client complains of intractable pain on rest, unexplained loss of weight, feeling generally tired or unwell. (Massage is sometimes given to alleviate pain, but only under medical supervision in particular circumstances.)

◎ Acute infectious disease and fever: if the client feels hot, feverish, is perspiring and generally unwell.

◎ Nausea: if the client is feeling sick or has a severe headache.

◎ Dysfunction or disorders of the nervous system: e.g. multiple sclerosis, strokes, Parkinson's disease etc, where muscles may exhibit increased tone (spasticity), which may be made worse by massage. These clients should be treated under medical supervision.

◎ Drink or drugs: massage must not be given to anyone under the influence of drink or drugs, as such clients may not be in control of their faculties.

◎ Inflammatory disease: when the client is in the active phase of any inflammatory disease such as rheumatoid arthritis or when any area is red, hot and swollen.

◎ Pregnancy: in the late stages of pregnancy; if the client is experiencing any problems with her pregnancy seek medical advice.

◎ Haemophilia: a condition of diminished or absence of blood clotting. Anyone suffering from this condition will bruise and bleed easily, and should not be massaged.

◎ Phlebitis and thrombosis: phlebitis is a painful condition where the lining of the vein becomes inflamed and may result in a clot forming on the vein wall, known as thrombosis. Any pressure applied to the vein or increase in the force of the circulation may dislodge the clot with potentially fatal consequences.

The danger of massaging a client with these conditions is explained previously. Massage of the legs is a definite contra-indication and it is safer not to massage any part of the body as there will always be a slight risk.

Local contra-indications to massage

Areas with these conditions should be avoided:

◎ **skin diseases or disorders**: these may be irritated or spread by the friction of the hands over the part or by the lubricant, e.g. eczema, psoriasis, acne, any skin infections such as pimples, boils, carbuncles, rashes, bites. See list on pages 120–122.

◎ **wounds, cuts and abrasions**: risk of infection and blood contamination

◎ **recent or extensive bruising**: small bruises can be avoided

◎ **recent haemorrhage** or bleeding in an area

◎ **recent scar tissue**: there is a danger of breaking down recently formed scar tissue. However, when the scar is completely healed (after about six months) massage may be given and is useful for stretching and loosening old contracted scar tissue

◎ **recent operations**

◎ **any burn, sunburn or wind burn** on the area to be massaged

◎ **large, lumpy or inflamed moles**: other areas may be massaged

◎ **warts or skin tags**: avoid these

◎ **bone fractures**: avoid until healing is complete; other areas may be massaged

◎ **metal pins or plates** inserted to support fractured bones: avoid the area

◎ **swollen, hot or painful joints**

◎ **recent sprains or muscle strains**: there may be damage to ligaments, tendons and muscle fibres; these must be allowed to heal before massage

◎ **any swellings, painful or inflamed areas of unknown origin**: massage is used to prevent or alleviate oedema (swelling in the tissues), but medical advice must be sought if there is doubt as to the cause of the oedema and whether massage is suitable

◎ **heart conditions**: because massage is thought to affect the rate of blood flow it may have an undesirable effect if there is a heart condition. Always seek medical advice if a client has heart problems. Stress-related heart problems may be helped by relaxing massage

◎ **high blood pressure**: although blood pressure varies with age, weight and fitness, some people have consistently high blood pressure. Medical advice should be obtained if such people request massage. Massage can frequently help, especially if the condition is stress related

◎ **low blood pressure**: again medical advice should be obtained before massage treatment is given. These clients may feel dizzy or faint if they sit up or get off the bed too quickly following treatment. Always supervise and give assistance if necessary

◎ **varicose veins, varicose ulcers**: any obvious, protruding varicose veins must be avoided. Massage proximal to the veins can help relieve the pressure

◎ **weak muscles with poor tone**: effleurage and gentle kneading movements may be used but wringing and all percussion movements must be avoided

◎ **epilepsy**: it is safe to massage controlled epilepsy, but always seek medical consent. Do not leave anyone suffering from epilepsy unattended in a cubicle or on the couch

◎ **diabetes**: some sufferers can be treated but, as tissue healing is impaired in these clients, great care must be taken not to damage tissues particularly of the lower leg and foot. Seek medical advice before treating

◎ **thin fragile skin**: older clients with thin, crêpy skin and poor muscle tone must be massaged with great care. Pressure should be kept light to moderate and plenty of lubrication must be applied to prevent further stretching the skin. All percussion movements, i.e. hacking, cupping, beating and pounding, should not be given

◎ **osteoporosis**: great care must be taken when massaging anyone with this brittle bone disease. Plenty of lubrication and light pressure must be used. Light effleurage stroking and kneading are suitable but all percussion manipulations must be avoided

If massage is contra-indicated tell the client gently, explain carefully and do not alarm her/him. Tell the client that it is for her/his own protection and that you will continue treatment when the condition has cleared or when medical consent is given.

Skin lesions, disorders and diseases

It is very important to examine the skin thoroughly before giving massage. The skin can be affected by many problems, which must be identified prior to massage. Some will have to be avoided whereas others may need medical referral. If you have to encourage a client to see the doctor, you must do so in a very tactful manner and not alarm nor offend the client.

Macule: this is a mark or discoloured patch that lies flat on the skin.

Papule: this is a small elevated pimple.

Vesicle: this is a very small scaly blister containing fluid (bulla is a large blister).

Milia/whiteheads: these are small plugs of sebum covered by the stratum corneum and look like tiny white spots.

Comedone: this is a blackhead: it is a plug of compressed sebum that is oxidised on the surface giving a black spot. Blackheads are very common. Advise proper cleansing routines and a healthy diet. If the condition is excessive and accompanied by pimples and pustules, then refer for medical advice. Avoid the area when massaging.

Seborrhoea: this is a skin condition caused by over-activity of sebaceous glands. The nose, forehead and scalp are very oily and shiny and the hair appears greasy. Avoid the area, as massage may further stimulate the activity of sebaceous glands.

Acne vulgaris: this is a chronic inflammatory condition of the skin generally appearing at puberty, but it may also be seen in adults. It is thought to be due to hormonal changes and over-activity of sebaceous glands. It may be found on the face, chest, back and across the shoulders. In severe cases the skin will be red and inflamed and covered with pimples, pustules and blackheads. As the problem progresses, cysts appear, which are red swollen lumps beneath the skin. Advise good personal hygiene, a healthy diet, exercise and drinking plenty of water. If the condition is excessive or troubling the client, seek medical advice. Avoid massaging over the affected area.

Rosacea: this is a chronic inflammatory condition found on the face. The skin is flushed and red due to dilation of blood vessels, and appears coarse with enlarged pores. Papules and pustules may develop. It is thought to be caused by intolerance to certain food or drink or over-exposure to extremes of climate. Tea, coffee or alcohol may exacerbate the condition as will exposure to sun and wind. These clients will usually be under medical supervision: if they are not, suggest medical referral. Do not massage over the area.

Sebaceous cysts: these are a swelling of the sebaceous glands under the skin, which form a lump (sometimes called a wen). They usually appear as a small lump on the scalp, neck or back. Do not massage over the area.

Urticaria (hives): these are itchy, red, raised wheals formed on the skin that can be caused by an allergic reaction to certain foods such as shellfish, strawberries etc. It is usually widespread; do not massage.

Eczema: this is an allergy that forms red, itchy, scaly patches on the skin, which may ooze. Do not massage over the area.

Dermatitis: this is inflammation of the skin and has many causes. It may be due to contact with a substance to which the person is sensitive. It may be caused by a reaction to specific drugs or exposure to irritants.

Psoriasis: this is a chronic skin disease that may affect small areas behind the knees or elbows or it may be found over the entire body. It results in reddish patches covered with silvery scales that continually flake away. It is non-infectious but affected parts should not be massaged.

Skin cancer: there are three types of skin cancer:

1. basal cell carcinoma

2. squamous cell carcinoma

3. malignant melanoma.

When examining the skin be particularly aware of small ulcerated spots or moles that change shape or change colour. Dark-brown raised patches of skin with uneven edges should be medically referred.

Naevus: this is an abnormality in the pigmentation of the skin and is often present at birth:

- Spider naevus: this consists of a central dilated blood vessel with small ones radiating from it – like a spider. Frequently found on the face. Avoid massaging the area as the blood vessels in the face may be fragile.

- Strawberry mark: this is an area of pink to red skin. Avoid the area.

- Port wine stain: this may be quite a large area of dark red to purple skin. Usually found on the face. Does not usually fade. Do not massage the area as capillaries are already dilated.

Freckles: *(ephelides)* small brown pigmented areas of skin that become darker when exposed to sunlight.

Chloasma: this is a light-brown pigmentation of the cheeks, nose and forehead. Usually occurs during pregnancy and disappears after the birth.

Vitiligo: this is a total loss of pigmentation of the skin. It starts as small white patches, which can join up to form quite large areas of white skin.

Papilloma: *(moles)* these are small growths on the skin that vary in size and colour. They may be pale to dark brown and may lie flat to the surface or be raised above the surface attached by a short stalk. There is a danger of trapping these with the fingers when massaging. Massage around the area, avoiding the mole.

Bacterial infections include:

Pustule: this is an elevated lump of skin containing pus: pustules often develop when hair follicles are infected by bacteria.

Furuncle or boil: this is an abscess under the skin filled with pus, which is caused by bacteria entering the skin, usually through a hair follicle. Boils can be painful and should be medically treated. Do not massage over the area.

Carbuncle: this is a collection of boils, which can be very painful and must be referred for medical treatment. Do not massage over the area.

Impetigo: this is a highly contagious bacterial infection of the skin. Usually located around the mouth, it begins as an itchy red patch that develops into pustules and further into flaky crusts.

It is usually found in children, but adults may also be affected. This condition should be medically treated. Do not massage anywhere near the area.

Viral infections include:

Warts: these are caused by a virus causing rapid cell division. Common warts are raised with a rough surface and are usually found on the hands. Plantar warts (verrucae) are found on the soles of the feet and grow inwards. They are painful upon pressure and should be referred for medical treatment. Warts are very contagious: avoid touching them and avoid working on clients if you have a wart. Do not massage over the area.

Herpes simplex/cold sore: this is caused by a virus living in the skin of the lips. It produces an eruption around the mouth that starts as an itchy red patch and develops into vesicles or a weeping blister, which then form a crust. It is very contagious. Do not treat the face of a client with cold sores.

Herpes zoster/shingles: is caused by a virus that attacks the posterior root ganglion of a sensory nerve. It may lie dormant until the body is under stress when it erupts and produces vesicles along the pathway of the nerve. This condition can be very irritating and the pain may be severe. Clients with shingles would normally feel too ill to come for treatment, which is contra-indicated anywhere near the area.

Fungal infections include:

Ringworm (tinea): this is a fungal infection and has different names according to the part of the body affected.

Tinea pedis, known as *athlete's foot*, is the most common: this infects the skin around and between the toes, forming red, itchy, scaly patches on the soles and between the toes. The skin may become sore, soggy and white. It is highly contagious. Do not treat the feet and cover them with disposable socks when treating other areas.

Maintain high standards of hygiene in showers, steam rooms etc to prevent spreading the infection.

Tinea corporis, known as ringworm, infects the skin all over the body. Red, round, scaly patches that spread outwards can appear anywhere on the body. Do not massage.

Tinea capitis: this infects the skin and hair shafts of the head. Greyish, scaly areas with short, broken hairs are found on the scalp. Do not massage.

Infestation by animal parasites

Pediculus capitis: this is infestation of the head: the louse obtains nourishment through blood sucking, causes intense irritation and lays eggs called nits among the hair.

Pediculus corporis: this is infestation by the body louse. It lives in clothing and sucks blood for nourishment. It causes intense irritation of the body.

Pediculus pubis: this is an infestation of the pubic hair by crab lice: causes intense irritation and sucks blood.

Fleas: these jumping insects suck blood and their bites appear as a collection of red pimples, which are very itchy. *In the salon, all linen must be boil-washed to prevent the spread of these infections and infestations. If you suspect that a client is infested, advise her/him to seek medical advice.*

Scabies: this is an infestation by itch mites. These are parasites that burrow into the skin around the wrists and fingers. It produces extreme irritation and is very difficult to eradicate. *Any clothing, bedding or towels used by a person with scabies must be burnt. Do not massage. Advise the client to seek medical advice.*

Contra-actions

These are conditions that may arise during the treatment that would indicate that the treatment must stop. During treatment be alert to any abnormal changes happening to the client which mean that you should not continue with the treatment. These conditions include:

- headache
- nausea
- vomiting
- profuse sweating
- restlessness and irritability
- feeling faint
- abnormal erythema
- the area becoming very hot and red
- stomach or any abdominal pain
- joint pain.

If any of these conditions arise, remove the lubricant, slowly place the client in the recovery position and allow her/him to rest for ten minutes or so. Stay with the client until s/he feels better. Allow the client to sit up slowly and rest in this position. If s/he is still causing concern, seek advice from the person responsible for first aid.

Compile a neat, clearly worded consultation card for use in the salon for massage clients.

❖ Referring clients to a medical practitioner ❖

Doctors are very busy people and do not have time to write letters in response to queries from therapists. It is therefore a good idea to compose a standard letter that explains the facts clearly and merely requires the doctor's signature. An example (for a female client) is provided on page 126. Doctors will not discuss a patient's medical condition with anyone other than the patient and they may not be prepared to sign such a letter. The client must then be advised to consult the doctor regarding the recommended treatment.

❖ Preparation for massage ❖

Preparation for massage involves the physical and mental preparation of the therapist and client as well as the preparation of the working area or room. The highest standards of health, safety and hygiene must be practised at all times. The massage therapist carries a heavy responsibility for protecting her/himself and the clients from the risk of cross-infection, infestation or any contamination by micro-organisms that cause disease. The therapist must be aware of, and practise, all the precautions and procedures necessary for protecting health and preventing the spread of disease.

Preparation of working area

◎ Ensure that the working area affords the client total privacy to change and receive treatment without being overlooked by others. The area may be a curtained section in a large salon, an individual walled cubicle or a small massage room. The therapist should ensure there is enough space to walk around the bed and work from all sides, and that there is room for a trolley with commodities, and a stool.

◎ The area should be warm, well-ventilated and draught free.

◎ It should be quiet, peaceful and free from distracting noise. Soft relaxing music may be played, but check with the client – some clients prefer to be quiet.

◎ The lighting should be soft and diffuse, not directed above the client and shining into her/his face.

◎ The colour scheme should be pale but warming, using pastel rather than harsh bold colours.

Address of salon

Date

Doctor's address

Dear Dr [*name*]

Your patient [*name*], of [*address*], has requested a [*type of massage, e.g. general body massage*] once a week. During my consultation with her, she mentioned that she has been suffering from [*illness, e.g. diabetes*] for some years. I would be very grateful if you would indicate her suitability for treatment by signing the consent below.

Thank you

Yours faithfully

[*Your name*]

....

Doctor's consent

I agree that the massage treatment you suggest would be suitable for this patient.

Signed

....

[*Doctor's signature*]

These factors encourage relaxation, which is of prime importance for massage treatments.

◎ The area must be spotlessly clean and tidy.

◎ Items required during the massage must be neatly arranged on the trolley shelf and protected with clean paper tissue or a small sheet.

◎ A plentiful supply of clean laundered towels and linen should be to hand.

◎ Extra pillows, small support pillows or rolled towels should also be to hand.

◎ Shower and toilet facilities for the client's use should be accessible and regularly cleaned.

◎ A hand basin or sink should be available for the therapist to wash her/his hands. Disposable towels or hot air dryers should be used to dry the hands. These must all be scrupulously clean.

◎ A lined bin should be to hand for disposal of waste.

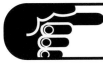 **Prepare a working area for massage.**

Selection of massage couch

Selecting and purchasing a massage couch can be difficult as there is a wide choice available. Selection is often based on the cost of the couch, but there are other important points to bear in mind when buying. Consider the following points:

◎ It must be wide enough for the clients to turn over easily and to feel safe and secure.

◎ It must be long enough to support the length of the body.

◎ It must be robust, secure and firm. It must not move or rock with the massage nor grate or squeak as this will disturb the client and prevent her/him from relaxing.

◎ It must be at the correct height for working. If it is too high the therapist will have to stretch to reach certain areas. S/he will not be able to use body weight correctly to apply the required pressure. If it is too low the therapist will have to bend over too much. This will cause shoulder and back problems. When standing upright next to the couch with the arms by the side, the couch should be just below the level of the wrist.

◎ The covering should be of smooth, washable material that is easy to wipe over and keep clean.

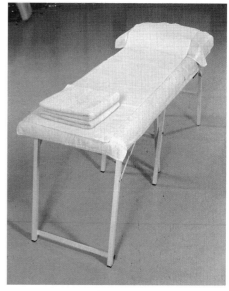

- If you need a couch that you can move from room to room or take on home visits then select the portable folding variety. Ensure that the legs are sturdy and that the hinges are secure and firm. Apply pressure sideways and to the top and bottom to test whether it shakes, rocks or stays firm.

If you are using the couch for other treatments, select from the multi-purpose varieties. The most useful couches are the adjustable height hydraulic varieties, but these are expensive and may be outside your budget. However, they are ideal for massage as the height can be adjusted to accommodate all types of client such as small and thin or large and obese. Some couches have a hole for the nose and mouth, to make positioning and breathing easier when lying prone.

Figure 3.2   A prepared treatment couch.

Preparation of massage couch

Prepare the couch before the client arrives.

- Cover the entire surface with a towelling or cotton sheet – the fitted types are best as they stay neat and tidy.

- Next cover this with a large bath towel or cotton sheet. This must be removed and boil-washed after each client and a clean one re-applied. Many salons and colleges use disposable paper sheets (bed roll) to save on the laundry – these are quite acceptable, but they can tear and crumple during the massage and may interfere with some movements.

- Use one or two pillows for the head. Cover these with pillow slips and then a towel.

- Fold two large towels and place them at the foot of the bed. These will be used to cover the client.

- Place extra pillows, large and small, and a rolled towel on the trolley for use if extra support is required during the massage.

Collect information from advertising leaflets on a variety of massage couches and select one that you feel would be suitable for you, giving reasons for your selection.

Preparation of trolley or table

◎ Select a trolley or table with a hard, smooth surface, free of cracks and easy to clean. Ensure that it is robust and sturdy so that it cannot be pushed over. Wheels are an advantage as the trolley may be pulled or pushed into a convenient position.

◎ Place the trolley near the massage couch so that all items will be to hand when required.

◎ Wipe the shelves with disinfectant of the correct dilution.

◎ Cover the shelves with paper sheets – fold under all edges for neatness.

◎ Arrange cleaned bottles and bowls neatly on this sheet. Always place commodities in the same order to ensure that they are easy to identify and reach when needed. Plastic baskets may be used to hold the bottles neatly. Clean these with disinfectant before loading.

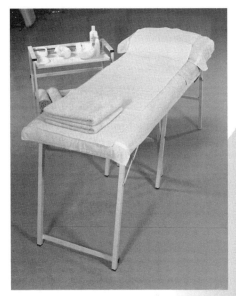

Figure 3.3   A prepared massage trolley.

◎ The following items should be laid out on the top shelf of the trolley:
   a) a bottle of cologne – for cleaning the skin if the client has not taken a shower
   b) a bottle of surgical spirit – to clean the feet
   c) a good quality oil, lotion or cream – used as a medium for the massage
   d) talcum powder or corn starch – these powders may be used instead of oil or cream as a massage medium. They work well for very hairy clients
   e) a bowl containing tissues and balls of cotton wool
   f) a bowl for placing the client's jewellery is sometimes used, but it is much safer to ask the client to place jewellery in her/his bag and place this under the couch.

◎ A bowl for waste, lined with clean disposable tissue, should be placed on a lower shelf, *or* a bin with disposable liner may be placed under the trolley. This is to avoid the risk of contamination of the commodities.

◎ Cover the shelf and commodities with a clean paper sheet when not in use. This will protect items from dust and dirt.

◎ At the end of each day, strip the trolley down. Wipe the shelves with disinfectant, clean all the bottles and bowls, then either store the commodities in a cupboard ready for use the following day or re-lay the trolley and cover.

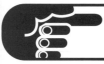 **Clean a trolley or table and prepare it for massage.**

Lubricants used for massage

Manufacturers produce a wide variety of oils, creams, lotions, gels and powders suitable for massage. The cheapest products are not always the most cost-effective, as you may need to use more of the product: the more expensive may go further. The massage medium should be selected to suit the client's skin type, and with experience you will develop your own preferences. It is important to try different types of lubricant when you are practising massage routines and also to try them on your own skin so that you know how it feels for the client.

Oils tend to offer the highest level of lubrication and are suitable for thin skin or hairy areas. Lotions and creams tend to be more nourishing and may have additives that are beneficial for dry skin. Gels and powders may be more suitable for oily skins because powder helps to absorb sebum and sweat, but if sweating is excessive, the powder, sebum and sweat may congeal to form a tacky mess. (If this happens, clean the area and use a more suitable medium.)

Massage can be performed without lubrication, and many manipulations where the tissues are grasped and lifted, such as picking up and wringing, are more effective when there is no lubrication and less slippage.

Neuro-muscular techniques are performed without lubrication because friction is required between the therapist's fingers and the skin in order to move underlying tissues.

Reasons for using lubricants

- reduce friction between the therapist's hands and the part
- improve the gliding movement of the therapist's hands over the part
- increase client comfort
- prevent dragging and pulling hairy skin
- prevent stretching loose, fragile skin
- nourish dry, scaly skin
- if used with appropriate essential oils, can produce psychological and therapeutic benefits.

Types of massage lubricants

Vegetable oils are the most widely used: these include almond oil, grapeseed oil, olive oil, corn oil, sunflower oil, wheatgerm oil, avocado oil, coconut oil, peanut (arachis) oil.

Mineral oils are also used: these include baby oil, liquid paraffin, cold cream.

Lanolin from sheep's wool is used as a base for some products.

Mineral oils are sometimes used but are not recommended as they are not absorbed easily and may block the pores in the skin. Less mineral oil is needed because it tends to lie on the surface of the skin for longer. (Remember to pour less mineral oil into the palm before massage.)

Vegetable oils are generally used, as these are absorbed into the skin and nourish it. These oils can be combined to provide the right consistency, e.g. a heavier oil such as olive oil can be combined with a lighter oil such as almond oil.

Aromatherapists add essential oils extracted from flowers and herbs to a carrier oil, but great care must be taken when mixing oils or adding essential oils, as their dilutions and prescription are specific.

Be cautious about mixing oils without adequate guidance and training from a qualified professional tutor.

Precautions

Lubricants may produce an allergic reaction in some clients. These reactions may range from abnormal reddening of the skin, raised wheals or a rash to very serious shock with fatal consequences. Many clients may be allergic to nut oils, in particular arachis oil from peanuts, which can produce anaphylactic shock, which results in rapid pulse, difficulty in breathing, profuse sweating and collapse. Check whether the client suffers from any allergies, during consultation and before massage. The client may not be aware that s/he is allergic to a product; it is therefore safer to avoid products containing nut oils. Be aware that essential oils have different properties and different effects, some of which may be harmful to your clients, e.g. oil of bergamot should not be used on parts exposed to sunlight as this oil increases skin sensitivity to ultraviolet rays. Knowledge of oils, their safe prescription, their dangers and dilutions is essential if you wish to mix your own. Otherwise buy your products from reputable manufacturers who are prepared to offer advice, give a detailed list of all the ingredients and discuss their preparations with you.

Read the manufacturers' instructions and list of ingredients before deciding on a product. Ask for samples to try before you buy.

Some vegetable oils can turn rancid and have a short shelf life: check this before you buy and buy small quantities only. Lubricants must be stored in containers with small apertures to prevent contamination by micro-organisms that could be transferred to you and the client. Self-dispensing plunge containers are the best.

Wash your hands before pouring the lubricant into the palm of one hand; do not pour too much and take care not to spill any, as this is wasteful and will make the floor slippery. Spread the lubricant between the palms of both hands to warm it before applying to the client.

Preparation of therapist

Before carrying out a massage therapists must prepare themselves physically, paying due consideration to high standards of professionalism and hygiene. They must also prepare psychologically and give due thought to the type of massage required.

Personal hygiene

◎ A daily bath or shower should be taken to maintain cleanliness of the skin, hair and nails, and to remove stale sweat odours.

◎ An antiperspirant should be used to prevent excessive sweating and the odour of stale sweat.

◎ Hair should be clean and neat; it should be kept short or tied back from the face. Hair must never fall forward around the therapist's face and shoulders or touch the client.

◎ Nails must be well manicured and kept short; nails should not protrude above the fleshy part of the finger tip. Massage movements cannot be correctly performed if the nails are long, and long nails may harbour dirt or bacteria. Nail enamel should not be worn as some clients may be sensitive to the product and an allergic reaction may result.

◎ Hands must be well cared for; they must be smooth and warm for massage. Therapists should protect the hands with rubber gloves when doing chores. A good-quality hand lotion should be used night and morning. Gloves should be worn in cold weather. Therapists should not massage with cuts or abrasions on the hands.

◎ Jewellery should be removed or kept to a minimum of wedding ring and small ear studs. Rings, bracelets and watches can harbour micro-organisms or can injure the client if dragged on the skin. Long earrings and necklaces may jangle, producing a noise that is disturbing to the client.

◎ Underwear and tights should be changed daily and washed in hot soapy water.

◎ White, short-sleeved overalls should be crisp, well laundered and changed frequently (e.g. every other day). The style should allow free unrestricted movement of the arms during massage.

◎ Feet should be well cared for and washed and dried thoroughly once a day, using foot powder if necessary. A clean pair of tights should be worn each day; support tights will help prevent tired legs and varicose veins. Well-fitting low-heeled or flat shoes without holes or peeptoes will protect the feet and avoid pressure points.

◎ Working uniform should not be worn out of the salon. Outdoor clothing worn to work should be changed in a cloakroom to prevent micro-organisms being brought into the salon.

◎ Therapists suffering from colds and infections should not treat clients if possible, but the wearing of a surgical mask will greatly reduce the risk of cross-infection.

◎ Therapists must wash their hands before touching a client and after cleaning the feet prior to the massage.

Psychological preparation

Preparing the mind enhances concentration and co-ordination and contributes to expertise and effectiveness of the massage.

◎ Develop a calm, tranquil but positive attitude. It is important to feel secure, confident and relaxed yourself as this is transmitted to the client both by your attitude and through your hands.

◎ Develop co-ordination between mind and body. The hands and body must move as a whole – think of your foot position, posture, arm/hand positions, speed, pressure and rhythm. Remember that massage is a skill that must be learned and requires constant practice to perform it well. It is very similar to learning to play a musical instrument.

◎ Develop sensory awareness, i.e. the ability to sense and visualise structures through the hands. Through the sensory receptors in the hands you learn to identify bony points, degrees of tone or tension in muscles, and variations found on different tissues and different clients. This ability only comes through practice and the experience of treating a variety of different types of client, e.g. young, old, thin, obese, well toned, poorly toned, tense or relaxed.

◎ Learn to synchronise speed, rhythm and depth so that these remain consistent throughout the treatment. These will vary depending on the effects required (see page 174). Maximum effectiveness of the treatment will occur only if these factors are co-ordinated.

Preparation of client

◎ Speak to the client in a polite and friendly manner.

◎ Maintain client privacy at all times.

◎ Take the client's outdoor clothes or show her/him where to hang them.

◎ Show the client the treatment area and shower room.

◎ Ask the client to undress and give her/him a robe or towel to wear.

◎ Ask the client to remove all jewellery and place it in a bag for safe keeping.

◎ Instruct the client how to use the shower.

◎ Bring the client back to the treatment area.

◎ Carry out a client consultation and discuss the treatment. As previously explained, the first consultation will be the longest but a short consultation should take place before every treatment. This will establish if there have been any changes and will provide feedback and results of the last treatment.

◎ Explain fully and ask if the client has any queries. Allow time for the client to discuss problems and ask questions, and answer these fully.

◎ If the client has long hair, ask her/him to tie it up, or provide a protective cover.

Lying

◎ Ensure that the client is safe at all times.

◎ Help the client onto the couch.

◎ Position the client correctly on the couch. A correct, well-supported position will ensure that the client is comfortable and will aid muscle relaxation. If the client is not well supported and comfortable, the muscles will be tense and will contract to hold the body parts. S/he will become restless and unable to relax and the massage will be ineffective. The position of the client must also allow the therapist to reach all areas easily without stooping or over-stretching.

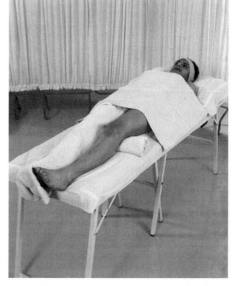

◎ Ask the client to lie centrally on the bed.

◎ Ensure that the client's body is straight.

◎ In the **supine** lying position (on the back) offer the client one or two pillows under the head for support. Another pillow placed under the knees will help to flatten the lumbar spine. Some clients like this knee support and it is particularly beneficial for those with back pain. This pillow must be fairly small and firm so that it does not hinder the leg massage.

Figure 3.4   Client in supine position for massage.

◎ In the **prone** lying position (face down) the head is usually turned to one side, with or without a pillow under the head depending on client preference. A pillow placed under the abdomen will round out the lumbar spine, which will make those clients with lordosis more comfortable. A small firm pad or tightly rolled towel can be placed under the ankles. This ensures that the anterior tibial tendons are not over-stretched. Alternatively the feet may just hang over the edge of the bed. The arms may be placed down along the body or bent and placed on either side of the head.

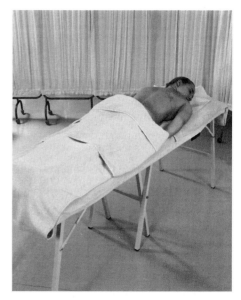

◎ Cover the client with two towels: one placed across the upper trunk from neck to waist; the other placed lengthways from the waist to the feet.

◎ Each part is uncovered when being worked on and then re-covered as the massage moves on.

◎ Always ask if the client is warm and comfortable.

Figure 3.5   Client in prone position for massage.

Sitting

Massage of the neck and upper back is frequently done with the client sitting. It is also a comfortable position for the pregnant client requiring massage for low back pain.

◎ Place a stool to the side or the end of a couch or table. Cover with a towel.

◎ Place one or two pillows on the couch and cover with a towel.

◎ Ask the client to undress, sit on the stool and lean forward onto the pillows.

◎ Ensure that the client is comfortable and well supported, with the arms and head resting on the pillow.

◎ Cover with a towel until the massage begins.

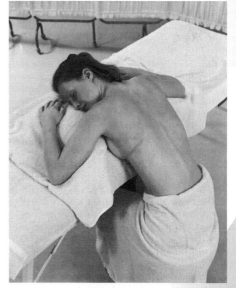

Figure 3.6   Client in sitting position for massage.

 Role play with a friend as the client.

a)   Position the client on the couch and prepare her/him for massage of the back.

b)   Position the client for a neck and upper back massage. Ensure her/his comfort at all times.

Use of heat prior to massage

Heating the tissues prior to massage enhances the effect of the massage. The application of heat will dilate the superficial blood vessels, and increase the circulation and metabolic rate. The warmth will relieve pain and tension, thus promoting relaxation. These factors will increase the effect of the massage that follows.

◎ Mild gentle heat may be given for 15–20 minutes.

◎ Any form of heating may be used, depending on client preference, suitability and availability; for example infra red, radiant heat, steam bath, sauna bath, hot pack.

◎ Heat should not be used if contra-indicated, nor in the treatment of oedema or acute injury.

(The principles of heat treatments can be found in *Body Therapy and Facial Work*, 1994, Mo Rosser, Hodder & Stoughton, p. 178).

QUESTIONS

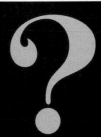

1. Give the meaning of the term 'contra-indication'.
2. List the reasons for the importance of a detailed consultation.
3. Name two contra-indications where medical advice should be sought.
4. Name two conditions where extra care should be taken.
5. Explain the factors you would consider when conducting an examination of a client prior to massage.
6. Explain briefly why high ethical standards are required in a massage therapist.
7. List ten factors that contribute to ethical behaviour.
8. State briefly how you would deal with a difficult client.
9. List the important factors that ensure high standards of personal hygiene.
10. Explain why the therapist's nails should be short and free of nail enamel.
11. Explain why outdoor clothing should not be worn in the treatment area.
12. Discuss the importance of psychological preparation prior to massage.
13. List the important environmental factors to consider when preparing the massage area.
14. Explain why the lighting in the working area should be soft and unobtrusive.
15. Give the factors that you would consider when purchasing a massage couch.
16. Explain how you would prepare the couch for massage.
17. List the items that must be arranged on the trolley prior to massage.
18. State why it is important to have a selection of oils and creams available.
19. Give the factors that must be considered when positioning the client on the couch.
20. Explain how you would position a client with lordosis to ensure maximum comfort.
21. Explain how you would position a client for massage to the neck and upper back.

4 | Classification of massage and the effleurage group

O B J E C T I V E S

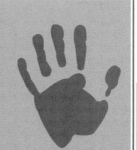

After you have studied this chapter you will be able to:
1. list the four main groups of massage
2. list the manipulations that belong to each group
3. explain the differences between effleurage and stroking
4. describe the techniques of effleurage and stroking
5. explain the effects of effleurage and stroking
6. explain when these manipulations may be used
7. perform effleurage manipulations on a client's back or leg
8. perform stroking on a client's back or leg
9. adapt effleurage to suit a variety of clients and conditions.

❖ *Classification of massage movements* ❖

The terminology used to describe and group massage movements has evolved over the centuries. There are differences in terminology from country to country and from school to school. The terminology used today is based on the Swedish remedial massage devised in Sweden by the physiologist Per Henrik Ling, and Dr Johann Mezgner of Holland. This has been modified over the years with input from French, German and British physicians and practitioners.

The names of the groups describe the action of the hands on the tissues. The four main groups are:

1 **effleurage:** where the hands skim over the surface of the tissues

2 **petrissage:** where the hands press down or lift and squeeze the tissues

3 **percussion or tapotement:** where the hands strike the tissues

4 **vibrations:** where the hands vibrate or shake the tissues.

Each of these groups may be further broken down into different manipulations that have their own technique and specific effects.

Table 4.1 Classification of massage movements

Group	Manipulations
Effleurage	Effleurage Stroking
Petrissage	Kneading Wringing Picking up Skin rolling or muscle rolling Frictions – circular or transverse
Percussion or tapotement	Hacking Cupping or clapping Beating Pounding
Vibrations	Vibrations Shaking

❖ *The effleurage group* ❖

The word 'effleurage' comes from the French verb *effleurer*, which means 'to skim over'. There are two manipulations within this group:

1. effleurage

2. stroking.

Although the two manipulations are similar, in that the relaxed hands move over the surface of the body, there are important differences to note. These differences lie in the direction of the strokes and in the differences in the pressure applied.

Differences between effleurage and stroking

◎ Effleurage must always follow the direction of venous return back to the heart and the direction of lymphatic drainage towards the nearest group of lymphatic nodes. Stroking may be performed in any direction.

◎ The pressure during effleurage may be light, moderate or heavy, but always increases at the end of the stroke towards the lymphatic nodes. The pressure of stroking is selected at the commencement and is maintained throughout. It also may be light, moderate or heavy pressure depending on the type of massage given.

◎ When performing effleurage, hand contact is maintained during the return of the stroke, although little pressure is applied. When performing stroking, the hands may maintain contact or may lift off the part on return.

❖ *Effleurage* ❖

As previously explained, effleurage is a manipulation where one or both hands moves over the surface of the body, applying varying degrees of pressure according to the type of massage being given. Effleurage will produce superficial effects when the pressure is light to moderate, but will produce deeper effects if the pressure is heavy.

Technique

1 Ensure that the client is warm and comfortable.

2 Take up a walk standing position with the outside foot forward: make sure you can reach all parts.

3 Remember to bend the front knee as the movement progresses and use body weight to apply pressure (pressure must not be applied through the arms and shoulders alone). Keep your back straight.

4 Ensure that your hands are warm, relaxed and supple – they must mould and adapt to the body contours.

5 The hands must move in the direction of venous return back to the heart, beginning distally and working proximally.

6 The strokes must be directed towards, and end at, a group of lymphatic nodes wherever possible.

7 The pressure should increase slightly at the end of the stroke.

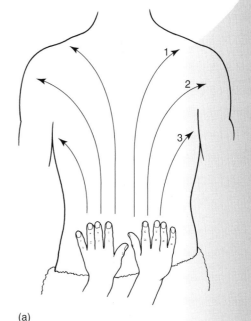

(a)

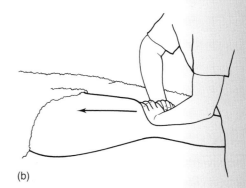

(b)

Figure 4.1   Effleurage (a) on back (b) on thigh.

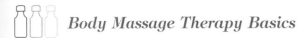

8 The hands maintain contact on the return of stroke but apply little pressure.

9 The movement must be smooth and rhythmical, with continuous flow and even pressure.

10 The whole of the palmar surface of the hand, fingers and thumb should maintain contact with the body in a relaxed manner. (Do not extend, abduct or link the thumbs, and do not spread the fingers out, as these habits will give uneven pressure.)

11 The hands usually work together with even pressure and rhythm. However, the hands may be used alternately when care must be taken to maintain an even pressure under each hand and to synchronise the flow and rhythm.

12 On small areas, one hand may work while the other supports the tissues. On very small areas such as the face, fingers or toes, the thumbs only may be used in a sweeping action.

Adapting effleurage

◎ Effleurage must be adapted to suit the client and the objectives of the treatment. For example, on the older thin client with poor muscle tone, the pressure will be light to moderate and plenty of oil will be applied. On a younger or fitter and well-toned client, the pressure can be deeper. A good covering of adipose tissue can take deeper pressure.

◎ For a relaxing massage, the effleurage will be rhythmical, slow and of medium depth. For a stimulating or vigorous massage, the effleurage will be rhythmical but faster and deeper.

◎ The effleurage performed at the end, to complete the treatment, should become progressively slower.

◎ When treating oedema, effleurage will *follow* kneading and squeezing movements – not precede them as is usual. The strokes will also change to begin proximally near the lymphatic nodes and work distally.

◎ When treating areas of cellulite the heavier movements of kneading and percussion are interspersed with effleurage, and the treatment ends with effleurage to increase drainage. Areas of cellulite are sometimes sensitive and painful to touch: check with the client if pressure is too heavy.

Deep effleurage

Heavier pressure is sometimes required to affect the deeper tissue and muscles. This does not mean the use of greater force but rather the more effective use of body weight. Deep effleurage is used for promoting relaxation in deep muscles and improving the local circulation. The manipulations are also used for athletic well-toned clients with muscle bulk.

Deeper effleurage movements include reinforced hand manipulations where one hand applies almost perpendicular pressure into the tissues reinforced by the other hand.

Effleurage with the forearm is another deep technique that is particularly effective over the large sheet-like muscles of the back.

Effleurage *du poing* uses the clenched fist to apply short stroking movements to particularly dense areas.

These techniques are also used to treat musculo-skeletal problems (see Chapter 9).

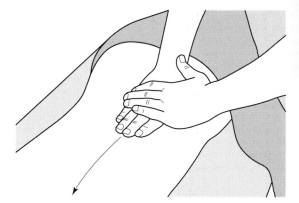

Figure 4.1c   Deep effleurage to the back using one hand to reinforce.

Effects

1 As the hands press on the tissues and move along they push the blood in the veins onwards. This speeds up the removal of deoxygenated blood and waste products from the tissues. Deep effleurage performed over muscles after exercise or any athletic performance will thus hasten the removal of lactic acid and relieve pain and stiffness. Effleurage will help the muscle to recover and return to normal function.

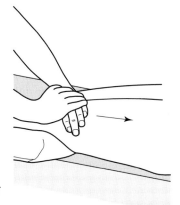

Figure 4.1d   Deep effleurage to the thigh.

2 As a result of increased venous drainage the blood flow through the capillary beds is speeded up. This increases the arterial blood flow, bringing oxygen and nutrients to the tissues more quickly. These factors improve the condition of the tissues.

3 The increased blood flow will increase the metabolic rate of the tissue cells, which also will improve their condition.

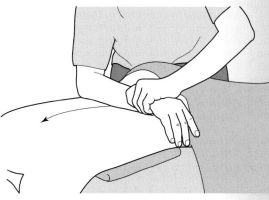

Figure 4.1e   Deep effleurage with the forearm over the back.

4 The increased blood flow and friction of the hands on the part will warm the area. This will aid relaxation and relieve pain.

5 The flow of lymph in the lymphatic vessels is also speeded up as the hands move along. This is directed towards the lymphatic nodes where it is filtered and then drained into larger vessels. Lymph removes large protein particles and tissue fluid from tissue spaces. Speeding up the drainage prevents stagnation of fluid in the tissues, which would result in oedema (swelling of the tissues). Effleurage and squeezing are manipulations used in the treatment of oedema.

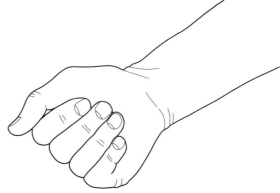

Figure 4.1f   Make a fist but keep the fingers flat.

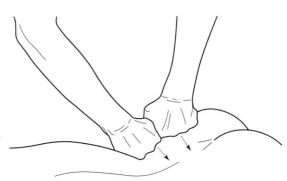

Figrue 4.1g   Deep effleurage du poing to the gluteal muscles.

6 The increased blood flow and dilation of capillaries in the skin will produce an erythema, which improves skin tone. The increased blood flow also nourishes the skin, improving its condition.

7 The cells of the stratum basale are stimulated and mitosis (cell division) increases. As more cells are produced they move upwards to the surface, improving the condition of the skin.

8 The movement and friction of the hands over the skin removes the dry flaking cells of the stratum corneum – thus desquamation is speeded up and the condition of the skin improves.

9 The oil or cream used as a medium nourishes and improves the skin.

10 The sebaceous glands are stimulated and produce more sebum, which keeps the skin soft and supple.

11 The warmth generated by massage stimulates the sweat glands, increasing the elimination of waste products.

12 Slow rhythmical effleurage has a soothing effect on sensory nerve endings in the skin, which will promote relaxation. However, if the pressure is very light or barely touching, the nerve endings will be irritated, or if the pressure is very deep the pain sensors will be stimulated. Both these effects will increase tension and should be avoided.

Uses

Effleurage is used:

1 to stimulate venous drainage and a sluggish circulation (to prevent varicose veins and varicose ulcers)

2 to stimulate lymphatic drainage and prevent or relieve oedema

3 to improve the condition of muscle tissue

4 to improve the condition and suppleness of the skin and produce an erythema

5 to promote relaxation using rhythmical slow movements of medium depth

6 to invigorate an area using rhythmical, fast movements with deep pressure

7 to remove waste products of fatigue following exercise, sport or athletic performance, thus relieving pain and promoting quick recovery

8 to help the warm-up of muscles prior to athletic performance (this must be used in addition, not instead of, a set of warm-up and stretch exercises). Warm-up exercise must always be performed prior to exercise sessions or athletic performance

9 as the first manipulation to enable the client to become accustomed to the therapist's hands and to aid client relaxation; as the last manipulation to conclude the massage

10 as a linkage movement to provide continuity and smooth transition between other massage groups

11 to spread the oil or cream used as the massage medium.

❖ *Stroking* ❖

Stroking is very similar to effleurage in that one or both hands moves over the surface of the body applying varying degrees of pressure, but there are differences as previously explained.

Technique

1 The therapist's stance depends on the direction of movement – walk standing (one foot in front of the other) if working top to bottom, stride standing (feet apart) if working from side to side.

2 The hands must be warm, relaxed and supple; they may mould and adapt to the contours of the body but this is not always so.

3 The wrists must be very flexible and loose.

4 The movement can be performed in any direction.

5 The pressure is selected at the commencement of the stroke and maintained throughout the stroke. This pressure may be light to moderate for a relaxing massage, or firm and heavy for a vigorous massage.

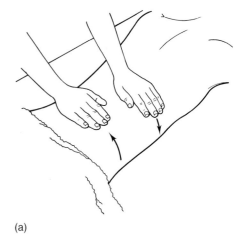

(a)

6 The movements must be rhythmical with continuous flow.

7 The hands may or may not be lifted off the part at the end of the stroke.

8 The whole of the palmar surface of the hand, fingers and thumb may remain in contact with the part, or the fingers only may be used.

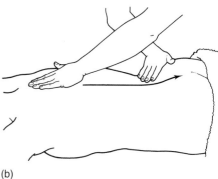

(b)

Figure 4.2   Stroking (a) across back (b) down erector spinae

9 The hands usually work alternately, one hand commencing a stroke as the other reaches the end.

10 The hands may work in opposite directions if working across the back, one beginning on the right side, the other on the left side, then crossing the back. Stroking is frequently performed from the nape of the neck to the base of the spine, or transversely across the abdomen, back or thigh.

Effects

Soothing stroking, performed slowly with light pressure:

1 soothes sensory nerve endings in the skin, which promotes relaxation

2 produces contraction of superficial capillaries, which will cool down an area

3 produces feelings of deep relaxation, which may induce sleep and help insomnia.

Stimulating stroking, performed vigorously with pressure:

1 stimulates sensory nerve endings, which counteracts feelings of lethargy and tiredness

2 produces dilation of superficial capillaries, which increases the circulation to the skin, giving an erythema

3 stimulates the sebaceous glands to secrete more sebum, which keeps the skin soft and supple, and the sweat glands to produce more sweat

4 may stimulate peristalsis and general movement of the contents of the colon. Use deep digital stroking of the abdomen in the direction of the colon.

Uses

Soothing stroking is used:

1 to soothe and relax a tense, nervous client

2 to help insomnia and promote sleep

3 to produce vasoconstriction on a hot, oedematous area.

Stimulating stroking is used:

1 to stimulate a lethargic client and arouse a tired one

2 to produce an erythema and warm up an area

3 over the abdomen to prevent or treat constipation.

 Role play the following with a partner.

◎ practise effleurage and stroking on each other

◎ comment on depth, speed, rhythm, continuity

◎ adapt effleurage for a relaxing massage, i.e. slow, deep, rhythmical

◎ adapt effleurage for a vigorous, stimulating massage, i.e. fast, deep, rhythmical

◎ always consider stance, posture and continuity.

Q U E S T I O N S

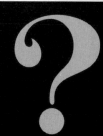

1. List the four main groups of massage.
2. List the movements (manipulations) in each group.
3. Give three different points of technique between stroking and effleurage.
4. Explain how you would adapt effleurage movements for the following clients:
   (a) the older, thin client
   (b) the young, fit, well-toned client.
5. Give six effects of effleurage.
6. List four uses of effleurage.
7. List six effects of stroking.
8. Give four conditions that would benefit from stroking.
9. Explain why the pressure of effleurage strokes should always be towards the heart.
10. Explain how effleurage strokes are adapted when treating oedema.

5 | The petrissage group

OBJECTIVES

After you have studied this chapter you will be able to:
1. list the five manipulations that belong to this group
2. subdivide and list all forms of kneading
3. describe the technique for each manipulation
4. explain the effects of each manipulation
5. explain the uses of each manipulation
6. identify manipulations for use on specific areas of the body
7. perform each manipulation on specified areas of the body.

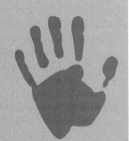

The word 'petrissage' comes from the French verb *pétrir* meaning 'to knead'. There are five manipulations in this group, but some can be further subdivided:

1 | kneading

2 | wringing

3 | picking up

4 | skin and muscle rolling

5 | frictions.

All the manipulations in this group apply pressure to the tissues, but each manipulation differs in technique. The true kneading manipulations apply pressure to the tissue and move them over underlying bone in a circular movement. However, other manipulations have evolved where the tissues are lifted away from the bone, squeezed and then released. Some of the manipulations in this group are quite difficult to perform and much practice is needed to perfect them.

❖ *Kneading* ❖

There are many forms of kneading. The terminology used for each one will tell you what should be done, so study them carefully.

→ **Palmar kneading**: this is kneading with the palmar surface of the hand. There are different forms of palmar kneading.

→ **Digital kneading**: this is kneading with the digits (i.e. the fingers) – the index, middle and ring fingers are usually used.

→ **Thumb kneading**: this is kneading with the thumbs.

→ **Ulnar border kneading**: this is kneading with the ulnar border of the hand (ulnar bone or little finger side).

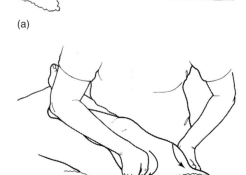

(a)

(b)

Figure 5.1   Palmar kneading (a) single-handed kneading (b) alternate palmar kneading.

Palmar kneading

Palmar kneading applies pressure to the tissues through the palmar surface of the hands and fingers, and moves the superficial tissues over the deep tissues.

The hands work in a circular motion, applying pressure on the upward part of the circle. This ensures that the pressure is applied in the direction of venous return to the heart and lymphatic drainage to the lymph nodes.

A variety of methods of palmar kneading may be used – selection depends on the area being treated.

◎ **Single-handed kneading**: one hand performs the kneading while the other supports the tissues on the other side. This is useful on smaller muscles such as triceps and biceps in the arm.

◎ **Alternate palmar kneading**: one hand works slightly before the other, resulting in alternate upward pressure. The hands are placed on either side of a limb (e.g. one on the abductors and one on the adductors of the leg) or they may be placed on the right and left side of the spine if kneading the back from the nape of the neck to the sacrum. One hand starts, then after half a circle the other hand begins producing alternate pressure upwards. This produces excellent mobilisation of the tissues.

◎ **Reinforced palmar kneading**: one hand lies directly on top of the other, reinforcing its movement. This produces very deep pressure, which is useful on large muscle groups such as the quadriceps, hamstrings, posterior tibials, and also on areas of dense adipose tissue over the hips, waist and sides of the trunk.

◎ **Double-handed kneading**: the hands work side by side, moving the tissues in a large circle with the pressure upwards. This is useful when covering large areas, e.g. from one side of the back to the other. It is also used over the quadriceps and hamstrings on very large thighs.

The petrissage group

Although these manipulations have different names according to the way the hands work, they are all methods of palmar kneading and the basic technique is the same for all.

Technique

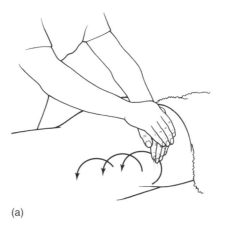

(a)

1 Stand in walk or stride standing, depending on the direction of work.

2 The hands must be warm, relaxed and supple – they must mould to the contours of the body.

3 The pressure must be directed upwards through the palms and fingers in the direction of venous return to the heart and the lymphatic drainage.

4 The pressure is applied upwards on each half circle and then released slightly to complete the circle.

5 The pressure must be firm enough to prevent skin rubbing. The flesh should move under the hands.

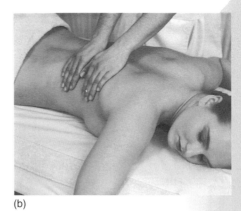

(b)

Figure 5.2   Palmar kneading (a) reinforced palmar kneading (b) double-handed kneading.

6 The heel of the hand must not dig into the part.

7 The movements must be smooth, rhythmical and with continuous flow.

8 The hands may work upwards and downwards in continuous sequence, or they may work in one direction and slide back, maintaining contact.

Effects

1 The alternate pressure and relaxation of the hands as they move over the area exert a pumping action on the underlying capillaries and veins. This speeds up the flow of blood through the vessels so that waste products are removed and fresh blood delivers nutrients and oxygen more quickly. This will improve the condition of the tissues.

2 The flow of lymph through the lymphatic vessels and towards the lymph nodes is speeded up in the same way. Thus, large particles of waste and tissue fluid are removed more quickly. This will reduce or prevent oedema.

3   Deep kneading has an effect on muscle tissue. The blood supply to muscles is improved. Waste products of fatigue are removed more quickly, which will reduce pain and stiffness, particularly following exercise or sport. Fresh blood brings nutrients and oxygen to nourish muscle cells. This improves the tone and condition of the muscles and aids recovery. Slow, deep, rhythmic kneading will increase the blood supply and raise the temperature of the muscle, giving a feeling of warmth that eases tension and promotes relaxation. If the massage is performed deeply and vigorously, the muscles are warmed and stimulated. Warm muscles contract more efficiently and are more elastic than cold muscles – they are therefore less likely to suffer injury. Vigorous massage may therefore be used prior to sport or athletic activities to enhance performance and prevent injury. It should be used in conjunction with, but not instead of, warm-up and stretch routines.

4   Kneading mobilises tissues, increasing their extensibility and flexibility. It loosens tight fascia and adhesions, allowing free movement of muscle bundles.

5   Deep kneading will press the tissues against the bone. This will stimulate the blood supply to the periosteum and the bone, resulting in an increase in delivery of nutrients to the bone.

6   Palmar kneading also affects the condition of the skin in a similar way to effleurage, i.e. the circulation to the skin is increased, producing hyperaemia and erythema. Therefore the condition and colour of the skin improves.

7   Sebaceous glands are stimulated to produce more sebum, which keeps the skin soft and supple.

8   The oil or cream used nourishes the skin.

9   The friction of the hands on the part and stimulation of mitosis increase the rate at which the cells of the stratum corneum are shed, which also improves the smoothness and condition of the skin.

10   Sweat glands are stimulated and excrete more sweat.

11   Kneading over the abdomen in the direction of movement of the contents of the colon will stimulate peristalsis.

Uses

Palmar kneading is used:

1   to stimulate a sluggish circulation and prevent varicose veins and varicose ulcers

2 to stimulate lymphatic drainage and prevent or relieve oedema

3 to improve the condition of muscle tissue and maintain tone and elasticity

4 to warm up muscles prior to exercise, sport or athletic performance (warm-up and stretch exercise must follow)

5 to remove waste products of fatigue following exercise, sport or athletic performance, thus relieving stiffness and pain and promoting fast recovery

6 to promote muscle relaxation

7 to produce a sedative and general relaxing effect

8 to mobilise tissues and improve extensibility, loosen tight fascia and adhesions

9 to improve the condition of the skin

10 to increase alertness and feelings of well-being and prevent lethargy, if the movements are performed briskly

11 to stimulate peristalsis and prevent or relieve constipation by kneading the abdomen in the direction of movement in the colon.

Digital and thumb kneading

Small circular movements are performed over small areas or small muscles using the pad of the thumb or the pads on the palmar surface of the first, second and third fingers. Again, the pressure must be applied in an upward direction, on half the circle, and then eased as the fingers come round and down. These digital movements are useful over the upper and middle fibres of the trapezius muscle, over the flexors and extensors of the forearm, down the erector spinae, around the colon, and over the pectoral muscles. Thumb movements are useful around the patella, over the anterior tibials, over the dorsum and sole of the foot, over the palmar and dorsal surface of the hand, and around the sacrum.

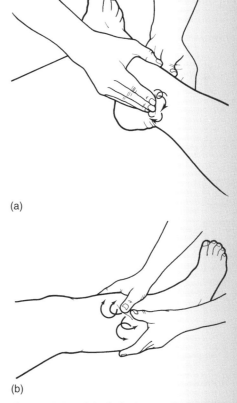

(a)

(b)

Figure 5.3 **(a) digital kneading**
(b) thumb kneading.

Technique

1 Select use of thumbs or digits depending on the area to be treated. Over smaller or confined areas such as the upper and middle fibres of trapezius, the thumbs are suitable but over larger areas such as over the length of erector spinae on either side of the spine, the digits are more suitable. Pressure may be applied alternately or together.

2 Place the thumbs or the digits on the area.

3 Select the depth of pressure according to the condition of the tissues and the type of massage.

4 Perform small circular movements with the pressure on the upward part of the circle. Ease the pressure on the downward part but maintain contact.

5 Do not hyper-extend the thumbs or fingers as the joints will be strained.

6 Avoid repeating the pressure over the same area as this may be painful for the client. Perform one circle and move smoothly and continuously to the adjoining area.

Ulnar border kneading

This is similar in technique, effects and uses to digital kneading but the ulnar border of the hand is used to obtain greater depth. The ulnar border of the hand is placed on the part and moved in circles. It is used mainly over the soles of the feet and around the colon in abdominal massage. When performed around the colon the pressure changes: the pressure is upwards over the ascending colon (on the right side); the pressure is across over the transverse colon; and downwards over the descending colon (on the left side).

Effects

1 The small kneading movements will increase the circulation to small localised areas, thus improving the condition of tissue.

2 They will mobilise localised areas and loosen adhesions.

3 Slow, rhythmical movements will promote relaxation and relieve pain over areas of tension and tension nodules.

4 They will increase lymphatic drainage in sluggish areas such as around the ankles.

Uses

Digital, thumb and ulnar border kneading are used:

1 to stimulate circulation to small areas as explained previously

2 to relieve pain and tension, especially over the trapezius and sacrum

3 to reduce fatigue and pain in the feet following prolonged standing

4 to break down or loosen adhesions.

❖ *Wringing* ❖

Wringing is a manipulation where the tissues are lifted away from the bone, and pushed and wrung from side to side as the hands move up and down. It must not be used on over-stretched muscles or those with poor tone.

Technique

1 The stance is usually stride standing.

2 The hands must be warm, relaxed and supple.

3 The tissues are grasped in the palm of the hand and held between the fingers and thumb (taking care not to pinch).

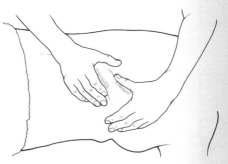

Figure 5.4 Wringing to the lateral aspect of the back.

4 The tissues are lifted away from the bone.

5 The tissues are moved diagonally from side to side by pushing the fingers of one hand towards the thumb of the opposite hand.

6 Keeping the tissues in the palm and lifted away from the bone, the hands move up and down along the length of the part, pushing the flesh from side to side. Do not pinch with the thumbs and fingers of the same hand.

7 The hands work up and down until the area is well covered and return to starting point.

Remember the fingers of the right hand work with the thumb of the left hand to press the flesh diagonally, then the fingers of the left hand move towards the thumb of the right hand. Wringing can only be performed over areas of loose or supple tissue that can be lifted away from the bone. Where tissues are firmly adhered to the bone, such as over the ribs or lateral aspect of the thigh where the fascia lata firmly binds the tissues, then wringing is difficult, ineffective and should be avoided.

Effects

1 The alternate squeezing and releasing action of the hands on the tissues again increases the circulation to the area, removing waste products and bringing oxygen and nutrients to the area, thus improving the condition of the tissues.

2 Tissue fluid is squeezed from tissue spaces and the flow of lymph is speeded up.

3 The increased blood flow will increase metabolism and stimulate and improve the condition of the tissues.

4 The increased blood flow will raise the temperature of the area slightly, which will aid relaxation and relieve pain.

5 This manipulation improves the elasticity and extensibility of the tissues; it stretches tight fascia and tight muscle fibres. It is very useful for easing tension and mobilising large muscle groups, especially before and after exercise.

6 When used over areas of adipose tissue, it stimulates and helps to soften the area.

7 It has a sedative effect on nerve endings when performed in a slow, rhythmical relaxing manner, but it stimulates the area when performed briskly and vigorously.

Uses

Wringing is used:

1 in conjunction with other manipulations to improve circulation and lymphatic flow

2 to warm tissues to ease tension and relieve pain

3 to improve the elasticity of skin and muscles

4 to stimulate, warm and soften areas of adipose tissue

5 to mobilise one tissue over another

6 to promote relaxation if performed slowly and rhythmically

7 to stimulate and invigorate if performed briskly.

❖ *Picking up* ❖

Picking up is also a manipulation where the tissues are lifted away from the bone, squeezed and released. It may be performed with one hand or with both hands. It must not be used on stretched muscles or those with poor tone.

Single-handed picking up: technique

This method is performed with one hand grasping the muscle.

1 The stance is walk standing.

2 Spread the thumb away from the fingers, i.e. abduct the thumb.

3 Place the thumb on one side of the muscle or group and the fingers together on the other side.

4 Grasp and lift the muscle in the palm of the hand, squeezing with the thumb and fingers (do not pinch).

5 Release the muscle and move the hand forward, pushing upward with the palm and web of the abducted thumb. Slight flexion and extension of the wrist accompanies this movement.

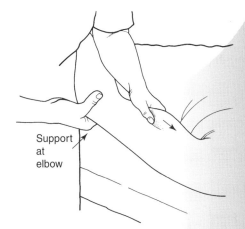

Support at elbow

Figure 5.5 Single-handed picking up of biceps.

6 The hand moves upwards in this manner, picking up, squeezing, releasing and moving on.

7 The hand may work up and down, or it may work up and slide back down.

8 Use the other hand to support the tissues.

Reinforced picking up: technique

For this method one hand is placed on the area as in single-handed work, but the other hand is placed over it to reinforce and provide more depth to the movement.

1 Place one hand (right if you are right handed) on the part, as explained in single-handed picking up.

2 Place the other hand over the top, with the thumb over the index finger of the underneath hand.

3 The hands then work together (like the wings of a bird) with the fingers of the right and left hand lifting, squeezing and releasing.

4 The elbows need to be fairly straight for this manipulation, as body weight is applied through the arms.

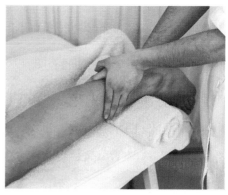

Figure 5.6   Reinforced picking up of gastrocnemius.

Double-handed picking up: technique

This is performed by two hands working in a synchronised manner up and down, usually on the large muscle groups of the leg or on adipose tissue at the sides of the trunk and hips.

1 The hands are placed on the area with the web of each abducted thumb facing towards each other, with the thumbs and fingers placed around the part and elbows out (abducted).

2 One hand starts lifting and squeezing the tissues (as before). On release of the tissues by this hand, the other performs the same action slightly above, maintaining the rhythm.

3 In this way the hands move up over the area in synchronised chugging movements.

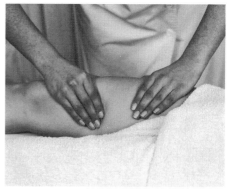

Figure 5.7   Double-handed picking up of thigh.

4 The pressure upwards is emphasised by the hand that is pointing and working upwards in the direction of venous return.

Effects and uses

The effects and uses of picking up are as for wringing.

❖ *Skin rolling* ❖

This manipulation presses and rolls the skin and subcutaneous tissues against under-lying bone.

Therefore it can only be performed where there is a bony framework underneath to work against. It is particularly effective when used transversely across the back, over the ribs or across the limbs.

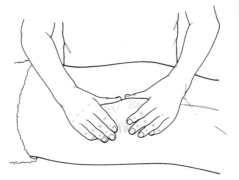

Figure 5.8   Skin rolling over ribs.

Technique

1 The stance is stride standing.

2 Place the hands flat over the area with the thumbs abducted.

3 Lift and push the flesh with the fingers towards the thumbs.

4 Roll this flesh, using the thumbs moving across towards the fingers.

5 Move smoothly onto a lower area and then work back.

Effects

These are mainly on the skin and subcutaneous tissue.

1 Skin rolling increases blood flow to the skin, thus producing an erythema.

2 The increased blood flow delivers nutrients and oxygen to the skin cells and removes waste products more quickly, thus improving the condition of the skin.

3 The oil or cream used nourishes the skin and improves its suppleness.

4 As the skin is moved over underlying tissues, its elasticity and suppleness is improved. This will help to soften established scar tissue.

5 The friction of the hands on the part aids desquamation.

6 Skin rolling stimulates and softens areas of subcutaneous fat.

7 It stimulates sebaceous glands to produce more sebum.

8 It stimulates sweat glands to excrete more sweat.

Uses

Skin rolling is used:

1 to improve the condition of the skin

2 to improve suppleness and elasticity of the skin

3 to soften and stimulate areas of subcutaneous fat

4 to soften and mobilise scar tissue

5 to induce relaxation if performed slowly

6 to stimulate and invigorate if performed briskly.

❖ *Muscle rolling* ❖

This manipulation lifts the muscle away from the bone and moves it from side to side in a rocking manner.

Technique

1 The stance is stride standing.

2 Place the thumbs nail to nail in a straight line on one side of the muscle and place the fingers over the other side.

3 Grasp and lift the muscle away from the bone.

4 Push the muscle with the thumbs towards the fingers, which give slightly as the muscle moves.

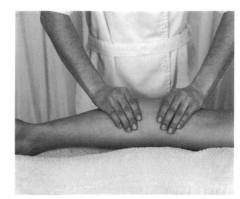

Figure 5.9   Muscle rolling on calf.

5 Push the muscle back towards the thumbs, using the fingers in the same way.

6 Push the muscle backwards and forwards, applying pressure into the muscle and using a rocking action.

7 Move along the muscle by sliding the hands.

Effects

1 Muscle rolling stimulates the circulation if performed briskly.

2 It improves lymphatic flow and drainage of tissue fluid.

3 It improves elasticity and extensibility in the muscle.

4 It releases tension in muscle fibres when performed slowly and rhythmically. It is particularly useful if pain is present in a muscle. Gentle muscle rolling can be tolerated and will ease the pain, allowing other movements such as effleurage or gentle kneading to be performed.

Uses

Muscle rolling is used:

1 to warm muscles and improve elasticity prior to sporting or athletic performance

2 to relieve pain and stiffness in muscles, particularly following sporting and athletic performance. This manipulation is particularly useful when muscles are very painful and sore and unable to tolerate any other pressure manipulations. The muscle is carefully grasped and very gently and rhythmically rocked to and fro until pain and tension are eased.

❖ *Frictions* ❖

These are very localised manipulations performed with the fingers or thumb. They may be applied transversely across muscle fibres or in a circular movement. They are deep movements performed with much pressure. The pressure may be selected at the commencement and kept constant throughout, as is usual with transverse frictions, or the pressure may get progressively deeper, as with circular frictions. The pressure must, however, be completely released before moving on to a new area. Frictions are performed on dry skin, free of oil or talcum powder, so that the fingers move the skin and do not slip over it.

Remember these are specialised movements, used when localised depth and pressure is required. They should not be confused with digital or thumb kneading, which applies constant upward pressure using a circular movement.

Fast stroking is also sometimes referred to as brisk friction because the hands do apply friction to the area, but this covers a large area and is not localised.

Circular frictions: technique

These are small circular movements performed by the fingers or thumb.

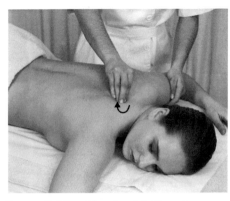

Figure 5.10 Circular frictions to tension nodules in trapezius.

1	The stance is usually walk standing.

2	Select and examine the small localised area where frictions are required.

3	Stroke it gently with the sweeping thumb or palm.

4	Use the thumb or the fingers: the middle finger is usually used to reinforce the index and ring fingers.

5	Do not hyper-extend any joints when applying pressure, as this will strain and damage the joints. Keep the fingers straight.

6	Circular frictions are performed in small circles, moving deeper and deeper into the tissues to a maximum depth, then released. Repeat three to four times over the same spot and then move to another area as required.

7	The fingers or thumb must not slide or rub over the surface of the skin, but the superficial tissues must move with the fingers over the deeper ones.

8	Areas requiring frictions may be tender and care must be taken not to cause unnecessary pain through excessive pressure.

9	Effleurage or stroke the area frequently between friction manipulations and at the end of the treatment.

Transverse frictions: technique

These are backward and forward transverse movements performed across ligaments or joints.

1	The stance is stride standing or walk standing.

2	Select the area requiring frictions.

3	Use the thumb or fingers as before.

4	Take care not to hyper-extend the joints, particularly those of the thumb – this is so easily done when pressure is applied.

5 For transverse frictions, the pressure is selected at the commencement and is maintained throughout the movements – it does not get deeper.

6 Place the thumb or fingers at right angles to the part, e.g. the ligament or muscle fibres, and move transversely across it, forwards and backwards six to eight times. Release and repeat.

7 Take care not to cause unnecessary pain by selecting too deep a pressure.

8 Effleurage or stroke the area frequently.

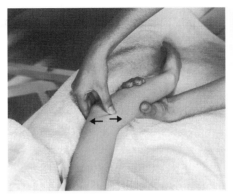

Figure 5.11   Transverse frictions to the extensor tendon.

Effects

1 Friction increases the circulation to localised areas, producing an erythema.

2 When friction is performed over ligaments and around joints the circulation to the area is increased, improving nourishment of ligaments and joint structures, and improving their function.

3 Movement of the tissues over one another will break down adhesions and mobilise fibrous tissue.

4 Deep frictions will break down and disperse fibrous nodules and ease fibrositic conditions.

5 Friction massage will improve the extensibility of old scar tissue and help to free scars from underlying tissues.

6 When performed on either side of the spine it will stimulate spinal nerves, producing feelings of invigoration.

Uses

Friction is used:

1 to increase local circulation and promote healing

2 around joints to loosen adhesions and improve movement

3 to stretch and loosen old scar tissue

4 to disperse tension nodules, found particularly in the upper and middle fibres of the trapezius

5 to increase the circulation and promote healing of chronic tendon strains, such as tennis or golfer's elbow

6 to stimulate and invigorate lethargic clients when performed along each side of the spine.

QUESTIONS

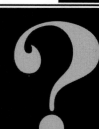

1. Name the five manipulations that belong to the petrissage group.
2. Explain what is meant by the following:
   (a) digital kneading
   (b) thumb kneading
   (c) ulnar border kneading.
3. List four types of palmar kneading.
4. Describe the effects of palmar kneading.
5. Give six uses of kneading.
6. State briefly how the tissues are manipulated in wringing.
7. Explain briefly why the temperature of the area is slightly raised when massaged.
8. Give six effects of wringing.
9. List six uses of wringing.
10. Explain briefly the difference between reinforced picking up and double-handed picking up.
11. Give the main tissue affected by skin rolling.
12. List six uses of skin rolling.
13. Explain the technique of muscle rolling.
14. Give one condition where muscle rolling is particularly effective.

The percussion and vibration groups

6

After you have studied this chapter you will be able to:

1. list the four manipulations of the percussion group
2. describe the technique for each manipulation
3. explain the effects of each manipulation
4. explain the uses of each manipulation
5. identify areas of the body where the manipulation would be effective
6. state conditions or areas of the body where these manipulations should not be used
7. perform each manipulation on appropriate areas of the body
8. state the difference between vibration and shaking
9. describe the techniques of vibration and shaking
10. list the effects and uses of vibration and shaking.

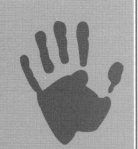

❖ *Percussion (tapotement) group* ❖

As their name suggests, all the manipulations of this group strike or tap the part. The hands are used alternately to strike the tissues with light, springy, rhythmical movements. When performing these manipulations, particular care must be taken to avoid bony prominences, ridges or areas where the bone is not well covered. They must not be performed on old or very thin clients, or those with loose, poorly toned muscles and little adipose tissue.

These manipulations are never used in a relaxing massage because they are too vigorous and stimulating.

There are four manipulations in this group, named according to the position of the hands and the way in which they strike the part:

1. hacking

2. cupping

3 beating

4 pounding.

❖ *Hacking* ❖

This manipulation uses the ulnar border of the hand and the little finger, ring and middle fingers to strike the tissues in a light, springy, brisk manner. The forearm must alternately pronate and supinate to allow the fingers to strike the part. The hands strike alternately.

It is important to avoid flexion and extension of the elbow joint as the resulting 'chopping' action is too heavy and powerful. This is a difficult manipulation to master and much practice is needed to perfect it. It can be practised initially on a pillow and the technique perfected before performing on a client. There are certain procedures to practise that will lead to correct and skilful technique.

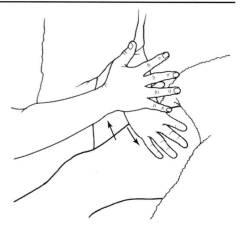

Figure 6.1   Hacking.

Technique

1 The stance should be stride standing, with the feet a good distance apart and the knees relaxed or bent, keeping the back straight.

2 Place the hands together with the fingers straight as in prayer, thumbs against chest.

3 Take the elbows away from the sides, i.e. abduct the shoulder joint. The wrists will now be extended at an 80–90° angle.

4 Place the arms parallel and just above the part to be worked on.

5 Supinate and pronate the forearm so that the little fingers strike the part lightly and then lift away.

6 Practise this action until the arms roll easily.

7 Now practise the whole procedure. Part the hands and strike the part alternately (remember to keep the elbows out and wrists extended).

8 Relax or slightly flex the fingers and, keeping the same action, strike the part alternately with the ulnar border of the little, ring and middle fingers.

9 Strike lightly, briskly and rhythmically with alternate hands.

10 Work up and down or across an area – cover thoroughly.

11 The hands may also diverge – the heels of the hand stay close but the fingers diverge forming a 'V' shape. This is useful over the upper fibres of the trapezius, below the nape of the neck.

Effects

The effects are similar for all the percussion manipulations, except that beating and pounding are heavier manipulations and produce deeper effects.

1 Hacking increases the circulation to the area, producing hyperaemia (increase in blood flow) and erythema (reddening of the skin).

2 It stimulates and softens areas of adipose tissue and is very effective on areas of hard fat and cellulite. Hacking over sensitive or painful areas of cellulite must be very light or omitted.

3 Hacking stimulates reflex contraction of muscle fibres and may increase muscle tone. It must be performed lightly and briskly. Because the other manipulations are not as brisk and sharp, they do not produce as great an effect.

4 The increased blood flow warms the area and increases the metabolic rate.

5 Hacking down either side of the spine stimulates spinal nerves and is generally invigorating.

Uses

Hacking is used to:

1 increase circulation to the area

2 warm an area

3 stimulate and soften areas of fat

4 invigorate and give a feeling of glow and well-being

5 stimulate muscles with poor tone.

❖ Cupping ❖

Cupping (also known as clapping) is performed using the cupped hands to strike the part alternately. The movements are light and brisk, producing a hollow sound.

Technique

| 1 | The stance is stride standing, as for hacking. |

| 2 | Make a hollow shape with the hand by flexing the metacarpo-phalangeal joints (knuckle joints). Keep the thumb in contact with the index finger. |

| 3 | Straighten the elbows – they may flex and extend slightly with the movement. |

| 4 | Place the hands on the part. |

| 5 | Flex and extend the wrist as the hands lift up and down alternately; keep the wrists loose and flexible. |

| 6 | Strike the part lightly and briskly with the fingers, part of the palm and heel of the hand. |

| 7 | The hands should clap the area, making a hollow sound. Avoid a slapping noise, which will occur if the hands are too flat. This will sting and be uncomfortable for the client. |

| 8 | Work up and down or across the area. Cover it thoroughly four to six times until an erythema is produced. |

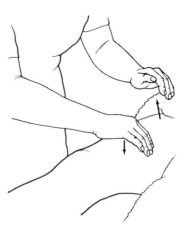

Figure 6.2   Cupping.

Effects and uses

The effects and uses of cupping are similar to those of hacking, but cupping is not as effective for stimulating muscle contraction.

❖ Beating ❖

This is a heavier percussion movement that is useful on very large heavy areas of adipose tissue, particularly over the buttocks and thighs. The manipulation is performed by striking the area with a loosely clenched fist. The back of the fingers and heel of the hands strike the part as the hands alternately drop heavily onto the area.

Technique

1 The stance is stride standing.

2 Loosely clench the fingers; keep the thumb against the hand.

3 Straighten the elbows.

4 Place the loosely clenched hands on the part so that the back of the fingers and heel of the hand lie in contact with the part.

5 Extend and flex the wrist and lift the arms slightly so that the hands fall alternately and heavily on the part.

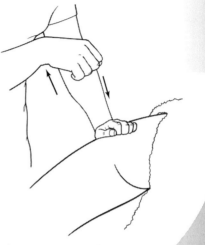

Figure 6.3   Beating.

6 Work up and down or across the area and ensure that you cover it thoroughly four to six times.

7 The movement should be brisk and rhythmical. The pressure can vary from light to heavy, depending on the required outcome and the type of tissue being worked on. Well-toned bulky muscles or a depth of adipose tissue (fat) will be suitable for heavier pressure.

8 It is usual to work with both hands striking the part alternately, but it is possible over small or awkward areas to use one hand only, supporting the tissues with the other.

Effects and uses

These are similar to hacking, but beating is heavier and is particularly effective in stimulating and softening adipose tissue.

❖ *Pounding* ❖

This, again, is a heavy percussion movement, performed by the ulnar border (little finger side) of the loosely clenched fist. The side of the hands strikes the part alternately.

Technique

1 The stance is stride standing.

2 Loosely clench the fingers.

3 Place the ulnar border of the hands on the part, with one hand slightly in front of the other.

4 Lift the front hand and strike behind the back hand as the back hand lifts off the part.

5 Continue to circle the hands over each other, striking the part alternately with each hand.

6 The movement should be brisk and rhythmical. The pressure can vary from light to heavy, depending on the desired effect and density of tissue.

7 Cover the area thoroughly four to six times, or until the desired erythema reaction is achieved.

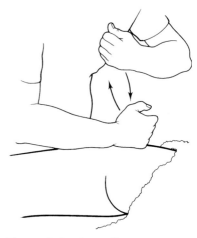

Figure 6.4   Pounding.

Effects and uses

The effects and uses of pounding are as for beating, cupping and hacking.

❖ *The vibration group* ❖

There are two manipulations in this group: shaking and vibration. Both produce vibrations or tremors within the tissues. Shaking is a much bigger, coarser movement and produces shaking of the muscle, while vibrations are fine movements that merely produce a tremor.

❖ *Shaking* ❖

This manipulation may be performed with one hand grasping and shaking the muscle while the other supports the part. It may also be performed with both hands working together, pushing in and out in a shaking action. This is particularly effective performed over the chest to loosen secretions and mucous in the lungs.

Technique

1 The stance is walk standing.

2 Support the part with the other hand so that the muscle is relaxed.

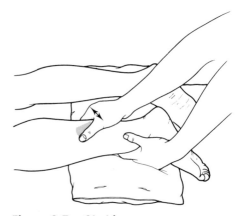

Figure 6.5   Shaking.

3 Grasp the muscle, usually towards its distal end. Lift it between the thumb and fingers, being careful not to pinch.

4 Shake the muscle gently from side to side. As the muscle relaxes, a greater degree of movement will be possible.

Effects

Gentle shaking will aid muscle relaxation, which will reduce pain and stiffness.

Uses

Shaking is used to relieve pain and stiffness in muscles, particularly after exercise or athletic performance.

Note: shaking of the chest to loosen secretions requires the correct positioning for drainage of lung secretions and is not covered in this book.

❖ *Vibration* ❖

This manipulation is usually performed with one hand. However, on large areas both hands can be used. The hand is placed over the area and vibrated either up and down or from side to side. The action produces vibrations in the underlying tissue.

Technique

1 The stance is walk standing or stride standing.

2 Support the part with one hand.

3 Place the other hand on the part.

4 Keep the fingers straight and the thumb adducted.

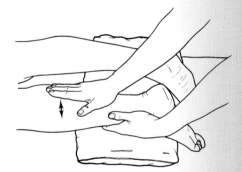

Figure 6.6   Vibration.

5 Vibrate the hand up and down or from side to side to produce a tremor in the tissues. The hand maintains contact throughout.

6 Avoid tension developing in the working hand, arm and shoulder.

7 The vibrations may be static and performed in one area only, or they may run or move over the part.

8 On small areas, and when very fine tremors are required, the finger tips only can be used to vibrate up and down or from side to side.

Effects

1 Vibration aids absorption of tissue fluid.

2 It soothes superficial nerves, which relieves tension and promotes relaxation.

3 When performed along the colon, it will relieve flatulence.

Uses

Vibration is used to:

1 stimulate sluggish lymphatic drainage

2 relieve tension and aid relaxation

3 relieve flatulence.

QUESTIONS

1. List the manipulations in the percussion group.
2. Name conditions when percussion manipulations would not be suitable.
3. Describe the technique of hacking.
4. Explain the effects of the percussion group.
5. Give four uses of this group.
6. Give one condition where beating and pounding are particularly effective.
7. Explain the effects of shaking and vibration on the tissues.
8. Give three uses of vibration movements.

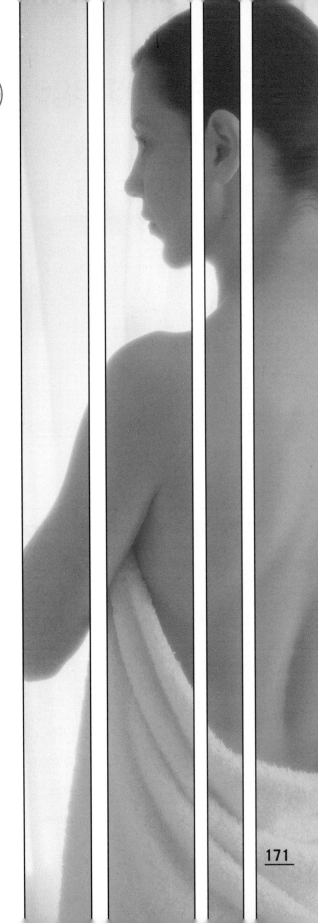

Part C

Massage routines and adaptations

7 Massage routines

After you have studied this chapter you will be able to:
1. give the approximate timing for each area when giving a general body massage
2. visualise the tissues in the areas being massaged
3. identify the principal lymphatic nodes
4. discuss the importance of continuity, depth, speed and rhythm and how they should be varied
5. select an appropriate form of massage to suit different conditions
6. perform a variety of manipulations on all areas of the body.

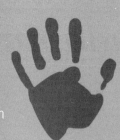

❖ *Basic guidelines* ❖

The timing of a body massage is usually one hour but may be longer. The order of covering the body is usually:

➤	right leg	7 minutes
➤	left leg	7 minutes
➤	left arm	5 minutes
➤	right arm	5 minutes
➤	décolleté	5 minutes
➤	abdomen	5 minutes
➤	back of legs	6 minutes
➤	back	20 minutes

172

Massage routines

These timings are approximate and will vary to suit client needs. More attention may be required on some areas than others. For example, if there were oedema of the ankles then a longer time would be spent on the legs.

Tension in the upper back would require additional manipulations and a longer time spent on this area.

Head massage is now very popular especially for reducing tension, and many salons and clinics offer head and facial massage as part of a full body massage.

Massage of the abdomen is frequently omitted. During the client consultation ask the client whether s/he wants the face and head massage included, and the abdomen left out. This must be decided before the treatment starts as it will affect the order and timing of the massage.

The conventional order of massage then changes so that the face and head massage conclude the treatment as shown below (reading *down* the columns).

→ back	→ left arm
→ back of left leg	→ right arm
→ back of right leg	→ abdomen
→ client turns	→ décolleté
→ front of right leg	→ face
→ front of left leg	→ head

These routines are for guidance only; the length of time you spend on each area can be adapted to suit the needs of the client. *The important point to remember is that there must be even coverage all over the body, and balance between the right and left sides. The right leg and left leg should receive the same number of manipulations at the same depth and rhythm; this also applies to the right arm and left arm. The client must not feel that any part has been neglected.*

When performing massage it is important to visualise mentally the tissues that the hands are moving over and to sense variations in tension or abnormalities through the hands. A knowledge of the anatomical structure of the area is therefore essential. The following text identifies the important structures, lists suggested massage routines and highlights areas where special care is needed. The lists of manipulations are suggestions only. Manipulations should be selected to suit the client and personal preference or expertise. There are, however, basic rules and guidelines.

1 **Comfort**: massage must always be comfortable. It must not hurt or injure the client, even the vigorous and stimulating techniques.

2 **Direction**: pressure must be applied in the direction of venous drainage towards the heart and the direction of lymphatic drainage to the nearest lymphatic nodes. (Do not pull back what you have pushed along as this is counter-productive.)

3 **Order**: begin with effleurage, follow with applicable petrissage manipulations then percussion if suitable, and complete with effleurage. Effleurage and stroking may be interspersed among any of the other manipulations.

4 **Continuity**: massage should be continuous – the transition between strokes should be barely perceptible. The hands should not be lifted off the area once treatment has commenced until that area is completed. Move smoothly from one stroke to another.

5 **Speed**: this must be selected according to the type of massage required – slow for relaxing, moderate for a general massage, and faster for a vigorous, stimulating massage.

6 **Depth:** this must be selected according to the type of massage, as described – moderate depth for a relaxing and general massage, deeper for a vigorous massage. Depth must also be adjusted to suit the client and the desired outcome of the treatment. For example, young, fit clients will take greater depth than older clients; well-toned clients will take greater depth than those with loose, flabby muscles or thin clients; obese clients or those with specific areas of hard adipose tissue will require greater depth. Those accustomed to massage generally prefer a deeper massage than new nervous clients. (Always ask the client if manipulations are too deep or not deep enough.)

7 **Rhythm:** this must be consistent regardless of the type of client. The rhythm is selected at the beginning of the massage and maintained throughout, e.g. slow rhythm for a relaxing massage, moderate for a general, and a faster rhythm for a vigorous massage.

8 **Stance:** protect yourself from strain and injury by adopting the correct posture. There are two standing positions used in massage:

a) walk standing (i.e. with one foot in front of the other) is used when massaging up and down the length of the body

b) stride standing (i.e. with the feet apart) is used when working across the body.

Always keep the back straight and the shoulders relaxed. Allow the knees to bend when necessary to apply body weight and to reach all areas. Increased depth and pressure must come from body weight transmitted through the arms, but not by pushing with the arms. Use a slight swaying body movement to achieve this. Keep the feet apart – this improves balance and provides stability, as it gives a wider base.

9 **Concentration**: maintain your concentration throughout the massage. Although massage movements become semi-automatic as expertise develops, it is still important to concentrate fully on the task in hand. Continuity and rhythm will suffer if there is a lapse in concentration, and this is transmitted to the client.

10 **Coverage**: cover the whole area thoroughly. Do not neglect small areas as this will result in uneven coverage.

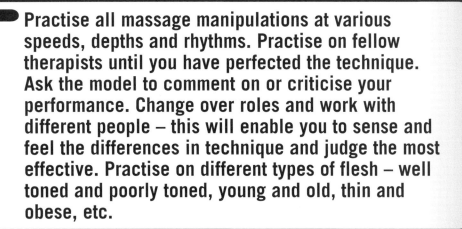

Practise all massage manipulations at various speeds, depths and rhythms. Practise on fellow therapists until you have perfected the technique. Ask the model to comment on or criticise your performance. Change over roles and work with different people – this will enable you to sense and feel the differences in technique and judge the most effective. Practise on different types of flesh – well toned and poorly toned, young and old, thin and obese, etc.

❖ *Leg* ❖

Bones

The leg contains the following bones:

◎ **femur**: thigh bone

◎ **tibia**: medial and larger bone of the lower leg

◎ **fibula**: lateral and thinner bone of the lower leg

◎ **patella**: small bone on front of the knee joint that allows the patella tendon of the quadriceps muscle to move smoothly over the knee joint

◎ **tarsals, metatarsals** and **phalanges** of the ankle and foot.

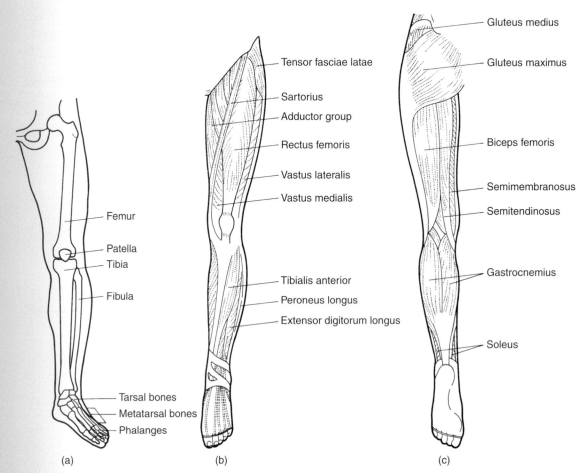

Figure 7.1   Anatomy of the leg: (a) bones (b) muscles (anterior) (c) muscles (posterior).

Joints

Table 7.1 Classification of leg joints

Name	Type	Movement
Hip	Ball-and-socket (synovial), formed by acetabulum of innominate bone and the head of the femur	Flexion, extension, abduction, adduction, rotation (medial and lateral) and circumduction
Knee	Hinge (synovial), formed by the condyles of the femur and the condyles of the tibia	Flexion and extension
Ankle	Hinge (synovial), lower end of tibia and fibula and talus	Dorsi flexion (foot up) and plantar flexion (point foot)
Intertarsal	Gliding (synovial) between tarsal bones	Inversion (turn foot in) and eversion (turn foot out)
Metatarso-phalangeal	Condyloid (synovial)	Flexion, extension, abduction, adduction and circumduction
Inter-phalangeal of toes	Hinge (synovial)	Flexion and extension

Muscles

Table 7.2 Classification of leg muscles

Name	Position	Action
Thigh		
Sartorius	Diagonally across front of thigh	Flexes the hip and knee joint
Quadriceps group (4)	Front of thigh	Large powerful group that extends the knee joint and keeps it straight when weight bearing
Rectus femoris	Front of thigh (superficial)	
Vastus medialis	Medial aspect of thigh	
Vastus lateralis	Lateral aspect of thigh	
Vastus intermedius	Front of thigh, deep	
Hamstrings (3)	Back of thigh	Work as a group to extend the hip joint and flex the knee joint
Biceps femoris		
Semimembranosus		
Semitendinosus		

(continued)

Table 7.2 (*continued*)

Name	Position	Action
Adductors (5) Adductor magnus Adductor longus Adductor brevis Pectineus Gracilis	Medial aspect of thigh	Work as a group to adduct the hip joint (pull inwards) and rotate it laterally
Abductors (3) Gluteus medius Gluteus minimus	Outer buttock region	Work as a group to abduct the hip joint and rotate it medially
Tensor fascia lata	Upper outer thigh	(Also tenses the band of fascia on the lateral aspect of the thigh)
Gluteus maximus	Large superficial buttock muscle	Extends the hip joint
Piriformis	Lies deep, across the hip joint	Abducts and laterally rotates the thigh
Lower leg		
Anterior tibials (3) Tibialis anterior Extensor hallucis longus Extensor digitorum longus	Antero-lateral aspect of lower leg	All dorsi flex the foot and invert it Extends the big toe Extends other toes
Posterior tibials (5) Gastrocnemius	Superficial calf muscle	Flexes the knee joint; plantar flexes the foot
Soleus	Deep to gastrocnemius and in the calf	Plantar flexes the foot
Tibialis posterior Flexor hallucis longus	Deep muscles of the calf	Plantar flexes the foot Flexes the big toe
Flexor digitorum longus		Flexor digitorum flexes the other toes
Peronei (3) Peroneus longus Peroneus brevis Peroneus tertious	Lateral aspect of lower leg	Dorsi flex the foot and evert it

Numerous small muscles lie in layers in the sole of the foot and between the metatarsals

Lymphatic drainage

There are two groups of nodes in the leg:

◎ **popliteal nodes**: behind the knee, into which the lymph from the lower leg drains

◎ **inguinal nodes**: in the groin, into which lymph from the leg drains.

Blood supply

MAIN ARTERIES

Blood is carried to the leg by the large femoral artery and its branches.

MAIN VEINS

Blood is carried from the legs by the great and small saphenous veins, the femoral vein and its branches.

Points to consider

◎ On the anterior surface of the lower leg the anterior border of the tibia, known as the shin, is protected only by skin and fascia (fibrous tissue). It forms a bony ridge down the front of the lower leg and must be avoided during massage as pressure on the bone may cause pain and discomfort. The anterior tibial muscles lie on the lateral aspect of this bone (towards the outside) and any kneading movements should be concentrated over this outer leg area.

◎ The medial and lateral malleoli on either side of the ankle joint must also be avoided, as must the patella on the front of the knee. Massage movements should be performed around these bony points, avoiding direct pressure.

◎ On the anterior surface of the thigh the large bulky quadriceps muscle and the adductors on the medial aspect are suitable for any of the massage manipulations. However, the upper third of the medial aspect, known as the **femoral triangle**, is a very sensitive area and must be avoided. The large blood vessels and nerves of the legs pass through this area.

◎ The lateral outer aspect of the thigh has a tight band of fascia, namely the fascia lata, passing from the muscle-tensor fascia lata down to the knee joint. This binds the tissues tightly, making it impossible to perform wringing, picking up or skin rolling on the outer thigh unless there is a depth of covering fat.

◉ The buttock and outer thigh area may be covered with adipose tissue (fat). In obese people the anterior and medial aspects of the thigh may also be covered. These areas can take the heavier manipulations of hacking, cupping, beating and pounding. Always ensure that you avoid the bony prominence of the greater trochanter on the outer aspect, just below and lateral to the groin.

Massage routine

The suggested massage routine for the leg is as follows:

◉ effleurage (front, sides and back)

◉ deeper effleurage over thigh

◉ alternate palmar kneading over abductors and adductors

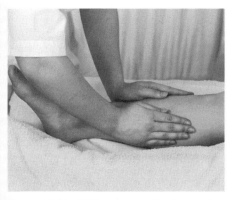

Figure 7.2   Effleurage to the lower leg.

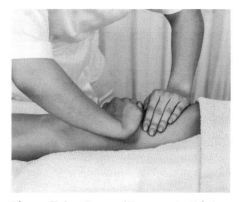

Figure 7.3   Deep effleurage to thigh.

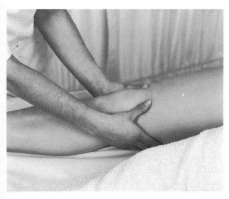

Figure 7.4   Thumb kneading around the patella.

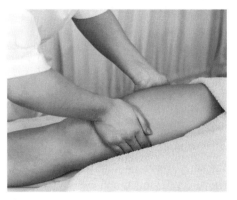

Figure 7.5   Alternate palmar kneading to abductors and adductors.

- reinforced or double-handed kneading over quadriceps

- wringing to thigh (medial to lateral and back)

- picking up – reinforced or double handed

- deep effleurage to thigh

- thumb kneading around patella

- effleurage to lower leg

- thumb kneading to anterior tibials (lateral to shin bone)

- alternate palmar kneading to calf

- stroking to dorsal surface of foot

- digital kneading around malleoli

- thumb kneading between metatarsals

- kneading to toes

- ulnar border kneading to sole of foot

- thumb kneading to sole of foot

- effleurage to whole leg.

Hacking and cupping are added to the thigh for a more invigorating massage, but not for a relaxing one.

Back of leg

This is usually performed after the abdomen, when the client has turned over, and before the back routine.

- effleurage to back of leg and buttock

- deep effleurage to thigh and buttock

- double-handed kneading to thigh and buttock

- reinforced kneading to top of thigh and buttock

- double-handed picking up to hamstrings

- deep effleurage to thigh and buttock

- effleurage to calf

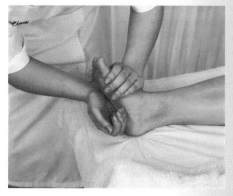

Figure 7.6   Ulnar border kneading to the sole.

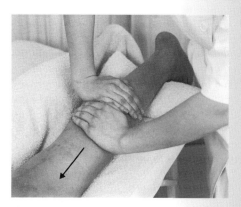

Figure 7.7   Effleurage of back of leg.

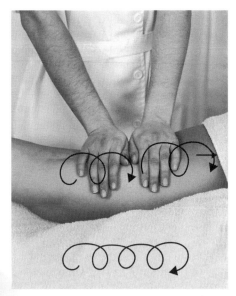 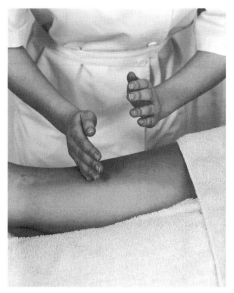

Figure 7.8   Double-handed kneading to hamstrings.   **Figure 7.9   Hacking to the thigh.**

- reinforced kneading to calf
- wringing to calf
- reinforced or single-handed picking up to calf
- effleurage to calf
- effleurage to leg.

Hacking, cupping, beating and pounding are used on the buttock for an invigorating massage and for treatment of cellulite.

❖ Arm ❖

Bones

The arm contains the following bones:

- **humerus**: bone of the upper arm
- **radius**: lateral bone of the forearm
- **ulna**: medial bone of the forearm
- **carpals**, **metacarpals** and **phalanges** of the wrists and hands.

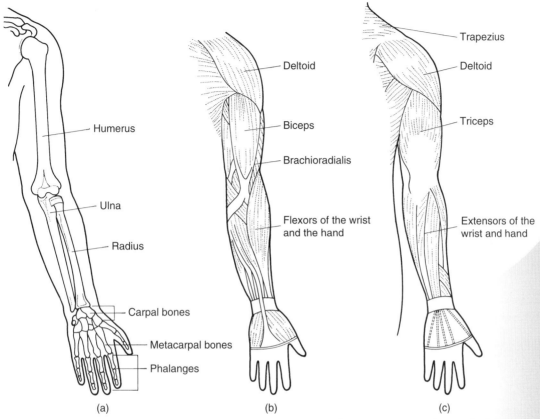

Figure 7.10   Anatomy of the arm: (a) bones (b) muscles (anterior) (c) muscles (posterior).

Joints

Table 7.3   Classification of arm joints

Name	Type	Movement
Shoulder	Ball-and-socket (synovial), formed by the glenoid cavity of the scapula and the head of the humerus	Flexion, extension, abduction, adduction, rotation (medial and lateral) and circumduction
Elbow	Hinge (synovial)	Flexion and extension
Radio-ulnar joint	Pivot (synovial)	Pronation and supination
Wrist joint	Condyloid (synovial)	Flexion, extension, abduction, adduction and circumduction
Metacarpo-phalangeal	Condyloid (synovial)	Flexion, extension, abduction, adduction and circumduction
Interphalangeal	Hinge (synovial)	Flexion and extension

Muscles

Table 7.4   Classification of arm muscles

Name	Position	Action
Deltoid	Covers the shoulder	Three sets of fibres: anterior fibres flex shoulder joint; middle fibres abduct shoulder joint; posterior fibres extend shoulder joint
Triceps	Posterior aspect of upper arm	Extends elbow joint
Biceps	Anterior aspect of upper arm	Flexes elbow joint
Brachialis and brachioradialis	Deep to biceps	Flex elbow joint
Flexors of the wrist and fingers	Many muscles lie in layers on the anterior aspect of the forearm	Flex wrist and fingers
Extensors of the wrist and fingers	Many muscles lie in layers on the posterior aspect of the forearm	Extend wrist and fingers

Small muscles of the hand lie in the palm and also form the thenar eminence on the thumb side and the hypothenar eminence on the little-finger side. Other small muscles lie between the metacarpals.

Lymphatic drainage

There are two groups of nodes in the arm:

◎ **supra trochlear**: at the elbow, drains the forearm

◎ **axillary:** in the axilla (armpit), drains lymph from the arm.

Blood supply

MAIN ARTERIES

Blood is carried to the arm by the axillary artery, the brachial artery, the radial artery and the ulnar artery.

MAIN VEINS

Blood is carried from the arm by the cephalic vein, the basilic vein, the brachial vein and the axillary vein.

Points to consider

◎ Deltoid is a muscle made up of three sets of fibres: one on the front of the shoulder joint; one over the top; and one on the back of the joint. Therefore, kneading of this muscle must cover all these areas.

◎ There is very little tissue on the lateral aspect of the upper arm and deep massage can be painful. Make sure that you are actually working in the correct area for the biceps and triceps. The biceps is easily found on the anterior aspect of the upper arm. The triceps is more difficult to find as the arm rotates laterally. It lies on the posterior surface, so find the olecranon process (funny bone) and work directly above it.

◎ When kneading on the forearm, remember that the flexors originate at the medial epicondyle, so on the anterior surface begin your kneading towards the medial side and work slightly across and down. On the posterior surface the extensors originate from the lateral epicondyle, so begin kneading from the lateral side. Knead around the styloid processes at the wrist.

Massage routine

The suggested massage routine for the arm is as follows:

◎ effleurage (front and back)

◎ alternate palmar kneading over deltoid

◎ single-handed kneading to triceps

◎ single-handed kneading to biceps

◎ wringing to triceps (if suitable)

◎ wringing to biceps (if suitable)

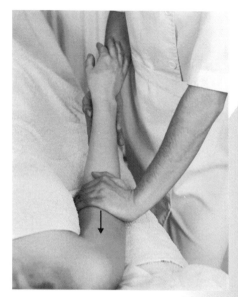

Figure 7.11   Effleurage of the arm.

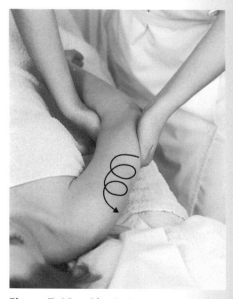

Figure 7.12   Single-handed kneading to triceps.

- ◎ stroking to upper arm (figure of eight)

- ◎ effleurage to forearm

- ◎ thumb kneading to flexors of wrist (anterior aspect)

- ◎ thumb kneading to extensors of wrist (posterior aspect)

- ◎ thumb kneading around styloid processes

- ◎ thumb kneading between metacarpals (dorsal aspect)

- ◎ kneading to fingers

- ◎ thumb kneading to thenar and hypothenar eminences and palm

- ◎ effleurage to arm.

Hacking may be performed on biceps and triceps for an invigorating massage.

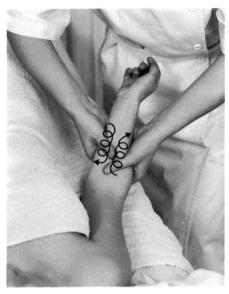

Figure 7.13   Thumb kneading to flexors of wrist and hand.

❖ *Chest and abdomen* ❖

Bones

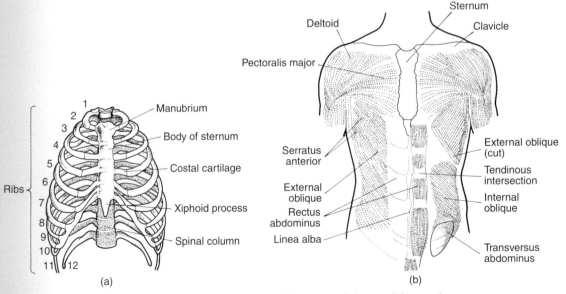

Figure 7.14   Anatomy of the chest and abdomen: (a) bones of thorax (b) muscles.

The chest contains the following bones:

◎ **sternum**: breast bone

◎ **clavicle**: collar bone

◎ **ribs**: 12 pairs.

Joints

Table 7.5   Classification of chest joints

Name	Type	Movement
Sterno-clavicular	Gliding (synovial) between the clavicle and sternum	Accompanies shoulder joint and girdle movements
Acromio-clavicular	Gliding (synovial) between the clavicle and acromion process of scapula	Accompanies shoulder joint and girdle movements

The ribs join the sternum via the costal cartilages and form a cage that protects the heart and lungs. There is no bony protection for the abdomen and its contents.

Muscles

Table 7.6   Classification of muscles of the chest and abdomen

Name	Position	Action
Chest		
Pectoralis major	Covers the chest	Flexes the shoulder joint and medially rotates it. Protracts the shoulder girdle
Pectoralis minor	Smaller and deep to pectoralis major	Holds the tip of the shoulder down during arm movements
Abdominal wall		
Rectus abdominis	Column of muscle, one on each side of midline	Flexes the trunk; one side working, side flexes the trunk
External oblique	Flat sheet of muscle passing obliquely down and in from ribs to pelvis and midline	Rotates the trunk to the opposite side; one side working aids side flexion of the trunk

(*continued*)

Table 7.6 (*continued*)

Name	Position	Action
Internal oblique	Flat sheet of muscle passing obliquely upwards and in from pelvis to midline and ribs	Rotates the trunk to the same side; one side working aids side flexion of the trunk
Transversus abdominis	Flat sheet of muscle passing transversely across the abdomen	Compresses the abdomen; used in all expulsive actions

Lymphatic drainage

There are three groups of nodes in the chest and abdomen:

◎ **axillary nodes**: in the axilla, into which lymph from the chest region drains

◎ **inguinal nodes**: in the groin

◎ **iliac nodes**: in the abdomen, into which lymph from the abdomen drains.

Blood supply

MAIN ARTERIES

Blood is carried to the chest region via the subclavian artery and to the abdomen via the common iliac artery.

MAIN VEINS

Blood is carried from the chest via the superior vena cava. Blood is carried from the abdomen via the inferior vena cava.

Points to consider

◎ Avoid pressure over the clavicle; work below. The clavicular glands that lie in the décolleté above and below the clavicle may become very tender in the pre-menstrual female and pressure should be kept very light. Always ask the client if she feels tender or sore when touched and adapt the massage accordingly.

◎ The abdomen has no bony framework for protection and the underlying abdominal organs will be affected by the massage. If muscle tone of the abdominals is poor, or if they are loose and over-stretched, then manipulations and pressure must be light. If the muscles are well toned or covered by layers of adipose tissue (fat) then deeper pressure may be used. Heavy percussion movements should be avoided over the abdomen and chest.

◎ Massage will stimulate peristalsis (the movement of alternate contraction and relaxation of the intestines) and is frequently used to aid movement through the colon. Pressure must therefore be applied in the direction of movement through the colon. This pressure must be upwards on the right-hand side of the abdomen over the ascending colon; from right to left along the transverse colon, just below the waist; and downwards on the left side along the descending colon. Make sure that the pressure is correct when kneading or stroking the colon.

Massage routines

The following are suggested massage routines for the chest and abdomen:

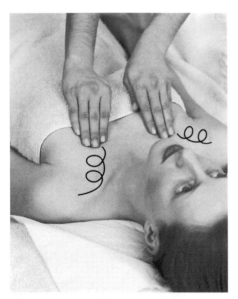

Figure 7.15   Digital kneading to pectoralis major.

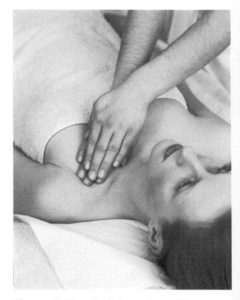

Figure 7.16   Reinforced stroking to the décolleté area.

Décolleté area

This area may be massaged before the abdomen, or if the routine changes to include the face and/or head, then the décolleté area can be included before the face massage as suggested later. The therapist's position will then change from the side of the couch to the head of the couch and the movements are adapted.

◎ stroking over area (right hand first, then left hand)

◎ effleurage around shoulders and back

◎ digital kneading to pectoralis major

◎ digital kneading to upper fibres of trapezius on back of shoulders

◎ reinforced stroking (figure of eight)

◎ effleurage

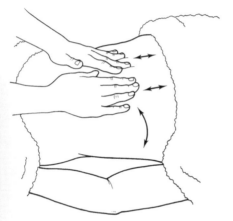

Figure 7.17   Effleurage to abdomen.

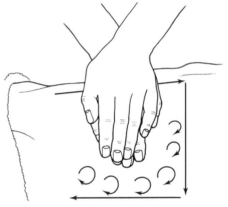

Figure 7.18   Digital kneading to colon.

Abdomen

◎ effleurage

◎ reinforced kneading to the waist

◎ wringing to the waist if suitable

◎ stroking over abdomen

◎ circular kneading around abdomen

◎ digital kneading around colon

◎ ulnar border kneading around colon

◎ stroking to colon

◎ effleurage

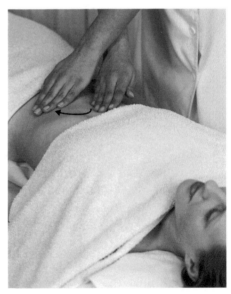

Figure 7.19   Circular kneading to abdomen.

❖ *Back* ❖

Bones

The back contains the following bones:

- ◎ **vertebral column**: made up of 26 separate bones in five regions – cervical (7), thoracic (12), lumbar (5), sacral (5 fused), coccyx (4 fused)

- ◎ **ribs**: 12 pairs of ribs form the thorax and articulate with the spine behind and the sternum in front

- ◎ **scapulae**: these lie on the upper back, one on each side of the vertebral column

- ◎ **innominate** or **pelvic**: these articulate with the sacrum behind, forming a ring of bone known as the pelvis. They join to form a cartilaginous joint called the symphysis pubis in front.

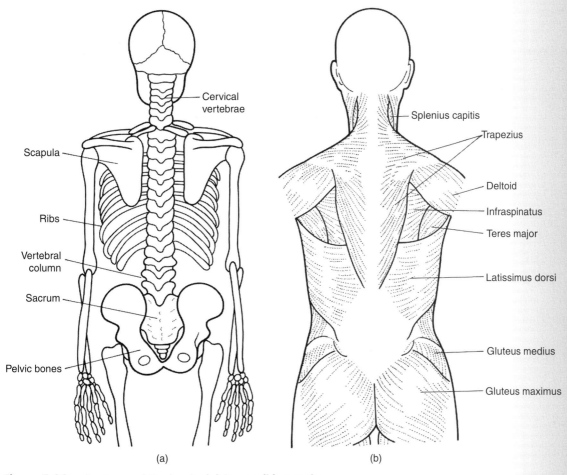

(a)   (b)

Figure 7.20   Anatomy of the back: (a) bones (b) muscles.

Joints

Table 7.7   Classification of back joints

Name	Type	Movement
Intervertebral	Cartilaginous, between the vertebrae	Very little movement between each pair, but considerable movement when spine moves as a whole. Flexion, extension, side flexion and rotation
Sacroiliac	Gliding (synovial) between the sacrum and right and left innominate bones	Hardly any movement; slightly increases during pregnancy

Muscles

Table 7.8   Classification of back muscles

Name	Position	Action
Trapezius	Covers the upper back	The upper fibres extend the head and elevate the shoulders. When one side is working it side flexes the head to the same side and elevates one shoulder. The middle fibres retract the shoulder girdle
Rhomboid major and minor	Lie deep to trapezius between the scapulae	Retract the shoulder girdle
Latissimus dorsi	Covers the lower back. From the lumbar region it passes upwards and outwards and inserts on the front of the humerus	Extends the shoulder joint and medially rotates it. Raises the trunk towards the arms as in climbing
Erector spinae	Lies deep to other muscles. Forms three columns from lumbar spine up along ribs to transverse and spinous processes to the cervical spine	Extends the trunk; one side working side flexes the trunk to the same side

(continued)

Table 7.8   (*continued*)

Name	Position	Action
Quadratus lumborum	Deepest muscle lying on either side of the lumbar spine	Extends the trunk; one side working side flexes the trunk to the same side
Splenius capitis	Deep to trapezius along the ligamentum nuchae into the occipital bone	Both sides working extends the head; one side working rotates the head to the same side
Splenius cervicus	Deep to splenius capitis	As above extends the head; rotates the head to the same side

Lymphatic drainage

◎ The upper back drains into the axillary nodes.

◎ The lower back drains into the inguinal nodes.

Points to consider

Before commencing massage it is important to examine the client's back carefully as many variations are found.

OBSERVE THE SPINE

◎ Is it straight or does it curve to the left or right indicating scoliosis?

◎ Is there a humped look in the thoracic region indicating kyphosis? An extra pillow may be required below the bust to improve contour and comfort.

◎ Is there a deep hollowing in the lumbar region indicating lordosis? An extra pillow may be required under the abdomen to level out the lumbar spine and improve comfort.

OBSERVE THE SCAPULAE

◎ Do they lie flat on the thoracic wall or does the medial border and inferior angle protrude backward, indicating winged scapulae?

◎ Are the scapulae level or is one higher than the other? This may indicate muscle tension in the

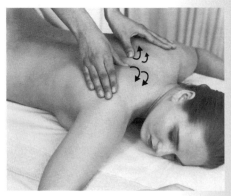

Figure 7.21   Thumb kneading between scapulae.

upper fibres of the trapezius or it may simply be the way the client is lying – adjust the client's position.

OBSERVE THE SKIN AND UNDERLYING TISSUE

◎ Are there any skin conditions that would make massage unsuitable (contra-indicated), e.g. extensive or pustular acne, large raised freckling, etc?

OBSERVE AND FEEL THE UNDERLYING TISSUES

◎ Does one area look raised? Is it hard and tense rather than soft and relaxed to touch? Are there painful, tender areas or nodules?

By observation, palpation and sensing through the hands in this way, you will build up a mental picture that will enable you to adapt your massage as necessary, e.g. avoid all bony prominences by working around them. Tense areas will require a slow, rhythmical, relaxing massage and tension nodules may require frictions or other special techniques, see Chapter 9. Extra work may be required over the upper and middle fibres of the trapezius. If there is pain in the lumbar region, the massage should be very light and gentle in that area.

Massage routine

The suggested massage routine for the back is as follows:

◎ stroking over back for palpating and sensing the tissues

◎ effleurage over back

◎ effleurage over trapezius (neck and shoulders)

◎ digital or thumb kneading to upper fibres of trapezius

◎ digital or thumb kneading from neck down between scapulae

◎ circular kneading around scapulae

◎ reinforced stroking around scapulae (figure of eight)

◎ alternate palmar kneading all over back

◎ reinforced kneading to waist

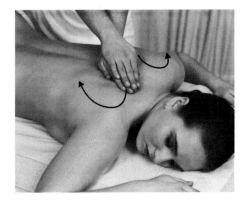

Figure 7.22   Reinforced stroking around scapulae.

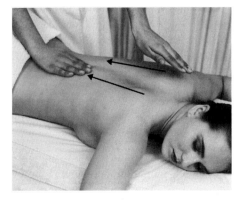

Figure 7.23   Stroking down erector spinae.

◎ wringing along hip, waist and side of ribs (if suitable)

◎ double-handed kneading over back (one side to other and back in four strips)

◎ transverse stroking over back

◎ thumb kneading to sacrum

◎ digital kneading down right and left erector spinae

◎ stroking down right and left erector spinae

◎ effleurage over back.

Light hacking and cupping over the back may be included for an invigorating massage.

❖ *Face and head* ❖

Bones of the skull

These include the cranial and facial bones.

Cranial bones

➤ One frontal bone

➤ Two parietal bones

➤ Two temporal bones

➤ One occipital bone

➤ One sphenoid

➤ One ethmoid.

Facial bones

➤ One maxilla (2 bones Fused)

➤ One mandible

➤ Two zygomatic

➤ Two nasal bones

➤ Two lacrimal bones

➤ Two inferior nasal conchae

➤ One vomer

➤ Two palatine.

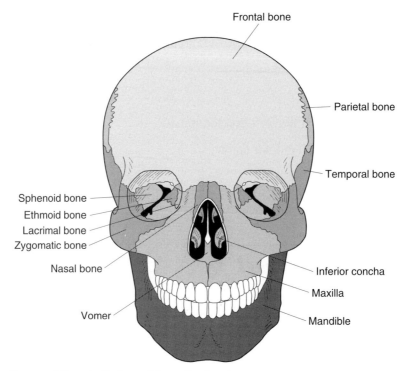

Figure 7.24a Bones of the skull viewed from the front.

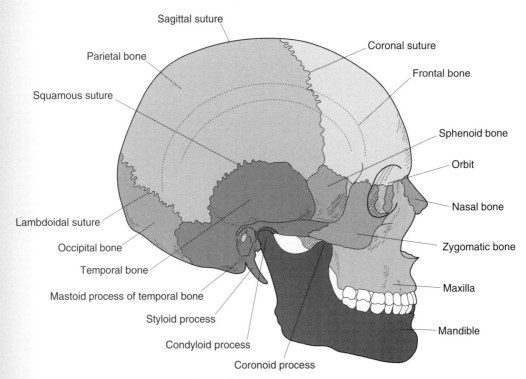

Figure 7.24b Skull viewed from the right side.

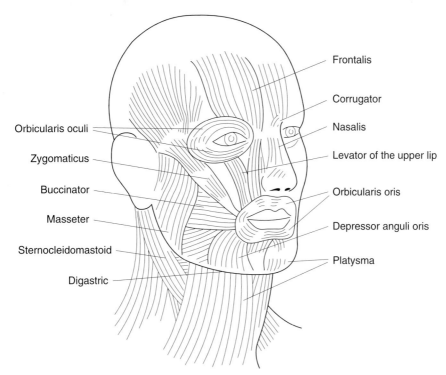

Figure 7.25a   Facial muscles.

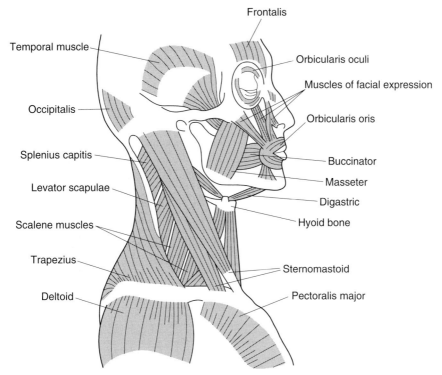

Figure 7.25b   Muscles of the face and skull, side view.

Table 7.9   Classification of facial muscles

Muscle	Position	Action
Occipito frontalis	Covers top of skull	Raises the eyebrows (surprise); wrinkles the forehead (frowning); moves the scalp
Corrugator	Between the eyebrows	Draws eyebrows inwards and down
Nasalis	Side of nose	Compresses the nostrils
Orbicularis oculi	Surrounds the eye	Closes the eye gently or tightly
Levators of the upper lip	Above the upper lip	Raise the upper lip
Zygomaticus	Above the corner of the mouth to zygmatic bone	Raises the corner of the mouth
Buccinator	Deep, horizontal in the cheek	Draws the teeth towards the teeth when chewing
Masseter	Between mandible and zygomatic arch	Raises the mandible to close the mouth
Depressor anguli oris	Below corner of the mouth	Draws corner of the mouth downwards
Orbicularis oris	Around the mouth	Closes and protrudes the lips
Digastric	Beneath the chin	Protrudes the jaw; depresses the mandible
Platysma	Covers the side and front of neck	Depresses the angle of the mouth; wrinkles the skin of the neck.

Lymphatic drainage

◎   anterior and posterior auricular nodes

◎   occipital nodes

◎   submandibular nodes

◎   superficial and deep cervical nodes

Blood supply
ARTERIES

Blood is delivered to the head via the *external* and *internal carotid arteries*.

VEINS

Blood is carried from the head via the *external* and *internal jugular veins*.

Décolleté and face massage

Decide during the consultation whether the face and head are to be included in the massage. Check for contra-indications in these areas. Female clients may not want their make-up and hair disturbed: make sure that you explain what is involved. If the face is included, cleanse it during client preparation. After the client has showered, position her/him on the bed, wash your hands and cleanse the face with a suitable cleanser followed by a toner. Clean the feet with surgical spirit; wash your hands again before starting the massage.

Technique

Stride standing at the head of the couch. Apply the lubricant to the face, décolleté region and around the back over upper trapezius.

1   Position the head in mid-line and press finger tips against the temples; hold for 5 seconds.

2   Slide the hands down the side of the face to the sternum.

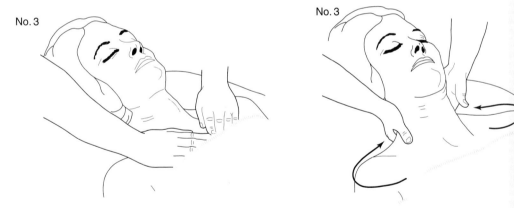

Figure 7.26a   Fingertips touching over the sternum.

Figure 7.26b   Sweeping effleurage over the pectoral muscles around the shoulders.

3   Finger tips touching over the sternum, press gently and begin sweeping effleurage out over the pectoral muscles, around the shoulders, over trapezius and the nape of the neck; return over the top of the shoulders to the sternum. Repeat 4–6 times.

4   Repeat these steps to the nape of the neck, then return around the back of the shoulders to the sternum. Repeat 4–6 times.

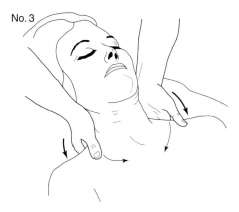

No. 3

No. 4

Figure 7.26c   **Return to sternum over top of shoulders.**

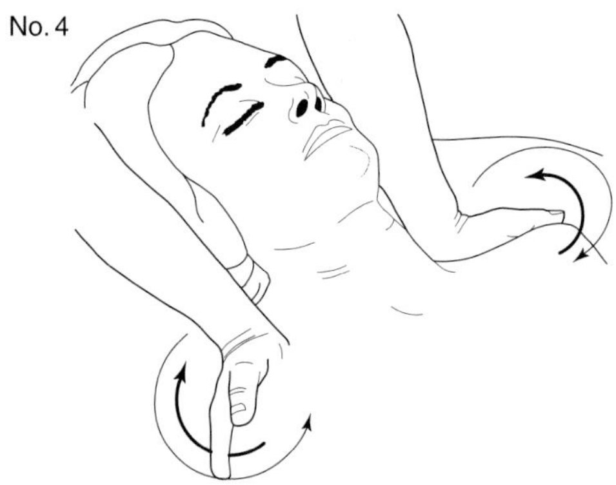

Figure 7.26d   **Return to sternum around the shoulders.**

5   Begin on the upper sternum below the clavicle, finger kneading to the pectoral muscles out to the shoulders; stroke around the shoulders and back to the sternum. Repeat a little further down each time until the area is covered (three strips are usually enough). Repeat the sequence 3 times.

6   Finger circular kneading to upper fibres of trapezius, begin at the shoulder and work in over the back and up the nape of the neck; slide back to shoulders and repeat 3 times.

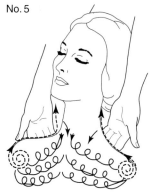

No. 5

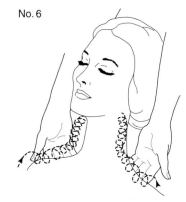

No. 6

Figure 7.26e   **Circular finger kneading in three strips to pectoral muscles.**

Figure 7.26f   **Circular finger kneading up the nape of the neck over trapezius.**

7   Knuckling over the pectoral muscles and knuckling over trapezius may be included depending on time constraints.

8   Repeat sweeping effleurage as just shown.

9   Place one hand over the clavicle and stroke up over platysma to the mandible; follow seamlessly with the other hand in a rollover manner; work from side to side over the neck.

No. 7

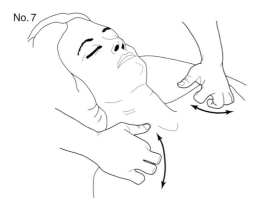

Figure 7.26g   Knuckling over the pectoral muscles.

No. 9

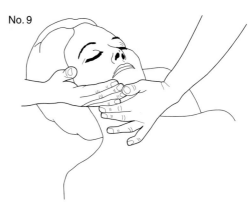

Figure 7.26h   Stroking over platysma, work from side to side.

10   Place middle and ring fingers in the centre under the chin, apply pressure upwards under jaw bone, move out slightly and repeat at 6–8 points.

11   Place index fingers touching above the top lip and middle fingers touching below bottom lip; draw fingers out and up to corners of mouth and slide back. Repeat 6 times.

No. 10

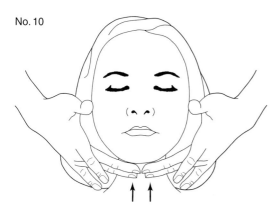

Figure 7.26i   Upward pressure under jaw line.

No. 11

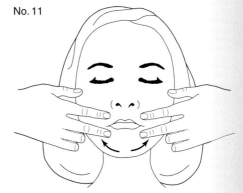

Figure 7.26j   Slide fingers out to corner of the mouth. Lift and slide back.

12   Place ring and middle fingers on the chin, circular kneading up over the cheeks to ear lobe; slide back to lips, repeat from corner of mouth to middle of ear, slide back to side of nose, repeat from nose to above the ear. Repeat the 3 movements 3 times.

13   Place ring and middle fingers at corner of the mouth, start circular kneading up naso-labial furrow to nose; slide the fingers up over the brow and back down to the mouth. Repeat 6 times.

No. 12

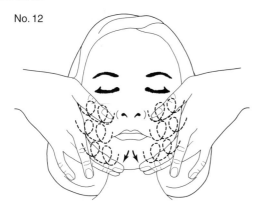

Figure 7.26k   Circular kneading over the cheeks.

No. 13

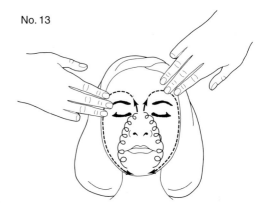

Figure 7.26l   Circular kneading to naso-labial furrow.

14   Place middle fingers on the temples, start light circular kneading under the eyes to the nose, stroke up the nose and across the brow back to the temple. Repeat 6 times.

15   Place finger tips on cheeks and tap lightly and upwards all over the cheeks. Cover well.

No. 14

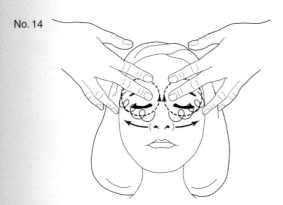

Figure 7.26m   Very light pressure, circular kneading below eye.

No. 15

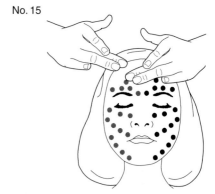

Figure 7.26n   Light tapping over the face.

16   Place the index and middle fingers on the forehead, pointing towards each other forming two V shapes; move the fingers towards each other and into the V; move the fingers in this way back and forth across the forehead. Cover well.

17   Place the right hand horizontally across the forehead and the other hand below it, begin slow stroking upwards with the right hand: the left hand follows seamlessly; cover the forehead from left to right as the hands roll over each other. Cover well.

No. 16

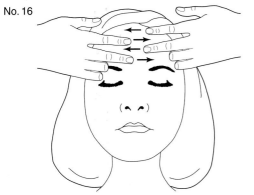

No. 17

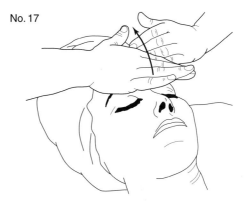

Figure 7.26o Index and ring finger on forehead, v-shaped movements in and out.

Figure 7.26p Stroking over the forehead.

18 Place the hands on either side of the face, fingers under chin; apply gentle pressure inwards and upwards to lift the face; be careful not to drag the skin. Hold and release slowly. Repeat 3 times.

19 Slide the hands up to temple, apply pressure, hold and slowly release.

20 Cover the eyes and press gently.

No. 18

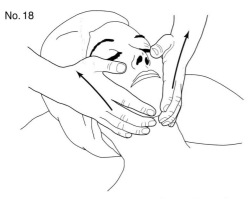

No. 20

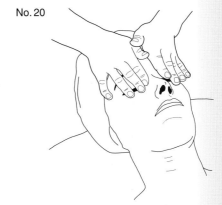

Figure 7.26q Apply pressure inwards and upwards to lift face.

Figure 7.26r Cover the eyes and press gently.

Head massage

Spread oil on to the hands and stroke through the hair from the roots to the ends.

1 Place the finger tips on the temples with the heel of the hand on the top of the head, press inwards, hold for 4 seconds and release. Repeat 4 times.

2 Place one hand across the forehead and the other across the back of the head over occiput, press inwards, hold for 4 seconds then release. Repeat 4 times.

3   Place the pads of the fingers on the head and perform circular frictions over the head. Cover well.

4   Place the pads of the fingers and thumbs on the hair line and stroke upwards slowly through the hair towards the crown, slide back and repeat. Cover well.

No. 3

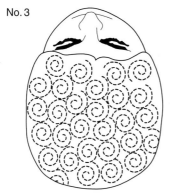

No. 4

Figure 7.27a   Circular frictions to the scalp.

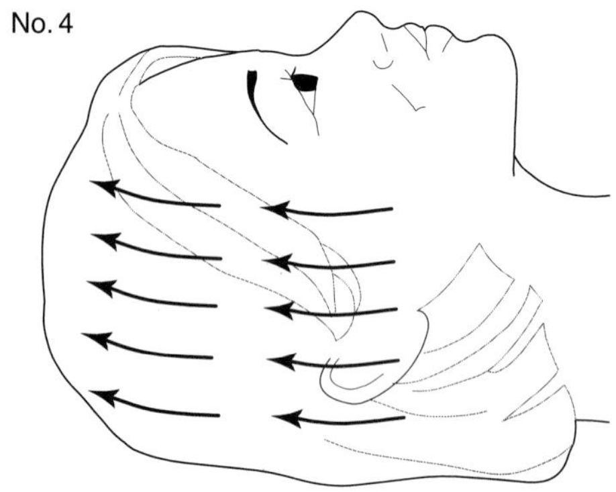

Figure 7.27b   Stroking upwards from hairline to crown.

5   Place the pads of the fingers in the hair and stroke with short brisk movements through the hair. Cover well.

6   Place the fingers at the base of the neck and perform circular kneading up on either side of the cervical vertebrae, then out towards the ears along the base of occiput; slide back. Repeat 3 times.

No. 5

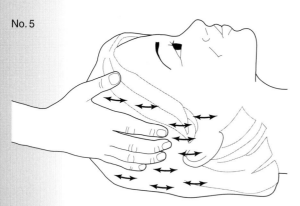

No. 6

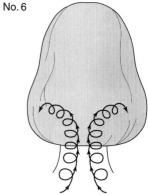

Figure 7.27c   Short brisk stroking over the head.

Figure 7.27d   Circular kneading to the neck and base of occiput.

7   Place the pads of the fingers over the scalp through the hair, move the scalp as the hands make large circular movements. Cover well.

8   Keep the fingers straight and tap very lightly over the head. Cover well.

Massage routines

No. 7

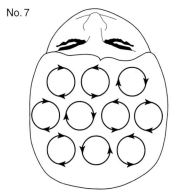

Figure 7.27e   Large circular kneading over the head.

No. 8

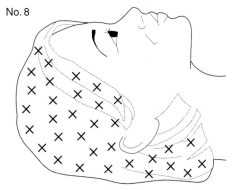

Figure 7.27f   Tap lightly over the head with pads of fingers.

9   Grasp the head with clawed fingers, then claw over the head from front to back. Cover well.

10   Stroke slowly and gently through the hair. Cover well.

11   Place fingers over the temples, press inward slowly, hold and release.

No. 9

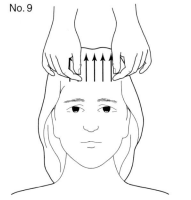

Figure 7.27g   Claw through the hair from front to back.

No. 11

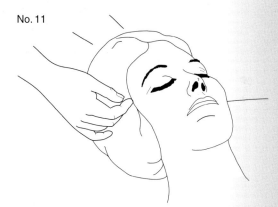

Figure 7.27h   Press temples.

QUESTIONS

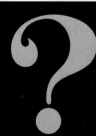

1. Explain the sequence of a body massage routine.
2. State how effleurage is incorporated into a body massage.
3. Explain how you would adapt depth, speed and rhythm for the following types of massage:
   (a) a relaxing massage
   (b) a general massage
   (c) an invigorating massage.
4. Give the two standing positions used in massage.
5. Name the large group of muscles on:
   (a) the front of the thigh
   (b) the back of the thigh.
6. Explain why it is difficult to perform wringing or picking up on the lateral aspect of the thigh.
7. Name the bony prominences on the leg, which must be avoided.
8. Explain why the heavier massage manipulations should *not* be performed over the abdomen.
9. Name two groups of lymphatic nodes in the leg and two groups in the arm.
10. Explain briefly how you would massage tight, tense muscles across the upper back.

8 Adapting massage for specific conditions

O B J E C T I V E S

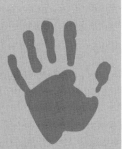

After you have studied this chapter you will be able to:

1. list the problems and conditions that may benefit from massage
2. explain the importance of psychological preparation prior to a relaxing massage
3. perform a relaxing massage for reduction of stress and tension
4. explain how visual and verbal feedback are obtained from the client
5. perform a massage to combat mental and physical fatigue
6. explain what is meant by the term 'oedema'
7. relate oedema to the function of the lymphatic system
8. select appropriate manipulations for the treatment of oedema
9. perform a massage to relieve oedema
10. describe the nature of cellulite and explain how it differs from soft fat
11. select appropriate manipulations for the treatment of cellulite
12. perform a suitable massage for the treatment of cellulite
13. discuss other treatments that may be used to treat cellulite
14. explain the advice you would give a client to combat cellulite.

❖ *Conditions that benefit from massage* ❖

During the initial detailed client consultation you will have established why massage is a suitable treatment for the client. The type of massage will vary depending on the desired outcomes of the treatment and on the age, physical and mental condition of the client.

It is important to be flexible and adaptable, and to avoid keeping rigidly to set routines. Manipulations and routines must be adapted to suit each client – some manipulations may be omitted while others will be used more extensively. Massage is beneficial for a variety of conditions and problems:

- ◎ to relieve stress and tension and promote relaxation

- ◎ to stimulate a lethargic client suffering mental and physical fatigue (to promote alertness)

- ◎ to relieve muscle fatigue, pain and soreness (post-performance or event)

- ◎ to relax very painful, stiff muscles

- ◎ to prepare and warm muscles prior to specific activities (pre-performance or event)

- ◎ to relieve or reduce areas of oedema (swelling)

- ◎ to stimulate and soften areas of cellulite

- ◎ to promote figure awareness during weight loss when used in conjunction with other treatments and diet

- ◎ to improve digestion and relieve constipation

- ◎ to improve the condition and tone of the skin

- ◎ to relieve stress for clients with certain heart and blood pressure conditions

- ◎ to relieve pain and stiffness in specific areas, particularly in the upper and lower back or to treat fibrositis.

❖ *Reducing stress and tension* ❖

Before commencing a relaxing massage it is important to prepare the mind as well as the body. The atmosphere created in the working environment must be quiet and calming. The area must be private, warm, well ventilated and free from distracting noises. The client must be positioned in a comfortable, well-supported position. S/he must feel safe and secure.

The therapist should adopt a relaxed, unhurried manner, speaking positively, calmly and quietly. Her/his movements should be smooth and gliding rather than sudden or jerky.

The client must be greeted pleasantly and made to feel cared for and cosseted. The procedure should be clearly explained and the client should be encouraged to ask questions, which must be answered immediately. S/he must be encouraged to discuss any problems or worries that may contribute to stress. A sympathetic but not patronising approach will reduce anxiety and help the client to relax. This is particularly important with new or nervous clients. Relaxation can be further encouraged by suggesting that the client empties the mind or concentrates on some pleasant visual imagery. Keep conversation to a minimum once the massage has started. Although most of these factors apply to most massage treatments, they are particularly important for relaxation and will greatly influence the effectiveness of the treatment.

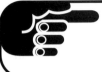 **List all the methods you would use to create a suitable atmosphere for promoting mental and physical relaxation.**

Treatment technique

The massage must be smooth, slow, deep and rhythmical. The transition between strokes should be continuous and barely perceptible. The tempo must be constant and unhurried. All the effleurage and petrissage movements in the suggested routines may be included, but percussion must never be included in a relaxing massage as the movements are too invigorating and stimulating.

You may wish to use more effleurage and kneading manipulations, repeating the movements until you feel the muscles softening and relaxing under your hands. You may need to concentrate and perform more manipulations on specific, identified areas of tension such as around the shoulder region, the upper or lower back or over the large muscle groups of the legs. Slow down each effleurage stroke at the end of the treatment.

Remember that it is very important to work calmly and unhurriedly, with constant, slow rhythm and medium depth. You must maintain your concentration throughout – you should relax mentally and physically as the massage progresses, but keep concentrating.

❖ *Combating mental and physical fatigue* ❖

For this type of client it is very important to create a stimulating atmosphere. Although the therapist must be caring and sympathetic, a positive, cheerful attitude is also required.

During consultation the client should be encouraged to discuss any problems and to establish reasons for the lethargy or tiredness. There are many factors that may cause the condition: stress at work or in the home; feeling overburdened or overworked; insufficient time for rest, relaxation or enjoyment; feeling unwell, suffering with headaches, migraine, insomnia or heavy and prolonged periods. There may also be psychological problems such as unhappiness, depression, feelings of low esteem or lack of achievement etc.

Encourage the client to seek solutions to the problems through changes in lifestyle, or to see a doctor if ill health is a cause.

> **List other reasons why clients may feel fatigued and lethargic.**

Treatment technique

Treatment for this type of client will be similar to that of a general massage. However, certain adaptations should be made. The massage movements will again be smooth, deep and rhythmical, but of moderate to brisk speed. The speed of the effleurage strokes may be increased with each movement. This is particularly important at the end of the treatment as it stimulates alertness. Note the difference from a relaxing or general massage, where the speed slows down towards the last stroke.

Petrissage movements should be deep and brisk. Light tapotement movements should also be included, unless there are contra-indications. These hacking and cupping movements are invigorating and may be performed over the quadriceps muscles, calf, hamstrings, buttocks, and very lightly over the top of the shoulders and along the back. Make sure that the client has a reasonable covering of flesh over the ribs and is not too thin, or tapotement will be painful and contra-indicated. Frictions performed along either side of the spinal column are also very effective, as they stimulate the spinal nerves. Complete the massage with brisk effleurage.

Discuss and plan the strategy for next time. Give home advice as appropriate. For example, you might suggest that the client should try to reduce her/his workload, allow time for rest, practise relaxation techniques, go to bed early some nights of the week, relax with a bath, and make time for enjoyment.

❖ *Relieving oedema* ❖

It is important to understand the structure and function of the lymphatic system before practising this massage (see Chapter 2).

Oedema is swelling of the tissues due to an accumulation and stagnation of tissue fluid in tissue spaces. Normally this tissue fluid is drained away through the blood vessels or lymphatic vessels. If these systems fail to drain the fluid away, it will remain in the tissue spaces. The amount of swelling can vary from slight puffiness to soft, mobile swelling that yields easily to pressure, or hard, consolidated, unyielding swelling of long standing. There are many possible causes of oedema:

- obstruction or blockage of the lymphatic system, such as an infected node

- interference in part of the system following surgery where glands may have been removed

➤ increase in the permeability of blood vessel walls or pressure within the vessels forcing fluid out. If this excess fluid cannot be removed quickly enough by the lymphatic system it remains in the tissue spaces

➤ lack of or poor muscle contraction, which normally acts as a pump and assists blood and lymphatic flow

➤ standing for long periods so that gravitational pull and lack of muscle contraction slow lymphatic drainage of the leg. Fluid collects around the ankle, which becomes puffy and swollen. The legs will feel tired and heavy

➤ systemic problems of the heart, lungs or kidneys.

Because massage speeds up the flow of blood in the veins and the flow of lymph in the lymphatic vessels, it is a useful treatment in the prevention and reduction of oedema. A brisk general or leg massage will be effective if oedema is recent, soft and due to gravitational effects. However, special techniques must be used if the oedema is of long standing, hard and consolidated, and the covering skin is shiny, thin and stretched. Great care must be taken not to break or damage the skin.

A squeezing movement is used to apply and then release pressure along the path of lymphatic flow. This alternating pressure technique forces the fluid out of the tissue spaces and speeds flow through the lymphatic vessels. It is important to drain and clear the proximal end first (i.e. the part nearest the lymph nodes). This ensures that fluid is not pushed into an already engorged area. The part must be elevated so that gravity assists the flow. Squeezing, kneading, effleurage and vibrations are the manipulations used.

Contra-indications

There are many causes of oedema and massage will not be suitable in all cases. Massage is contra-indicated if the oedema is due to the following conditions:

◎ disease of the heart, lungs or kidney

◎ acute injury

◎ deep vein thrombosis or phlebitis

◎ damage to the lymph glands following infection, surgery or radiotherapy.

Treatment technique
Oedematous leg

1 Prepare the client as for a general massage. Make sure that all restrictive clothing is removed and that there is no tight elastic if underwear is not removed.

2   Place the client in the supine position (face up). Make sure that the legs lie on the elevating end of the couch.

3   Elevate the leg to between 30° and 45° from the horizontal by raising the end of the bed if possible, or by using an arrangement of firm pillows. Make sure that the lymphatic nodes in the groin are neither stretched nor compressed.

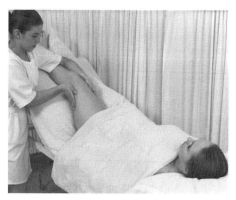

4   The legs must be allowed to drain in this position for half to one hour (you may massage other areas during this time). Massaging the abdomen can increase the effectiveness of the following leg massage. This is because lymph flow through the abdominal vessels, iliac nodes and lymphatic ducts is stimulated and drained away, reducing backward pressure. Deep breathing is also beneficial because, as the client breathes in and out, the pressure within the thoracic and abdominal cavities increases and decreases. The alternating high to low pressure acts as a pump, moving fluid along; this also reduces backward pressure.

Figure 8.1   **Position of client with leg in elevation.**

5   Examine the leg carefully before starting the massage. Check the skin and the degree of hardness of the oedema (does it 'pit' easily under pressure and refill quickly or slowly?). This will give some indication of how much pressure can be applied. If it is hard and unyielding, start with lighter pressure.

6   Take up a walk standing stance, level with the knee.

7   Imagine that you are pushing fluid through a tube or many tubes. To be effective, pressure must be applied to all the surfaces of the tube.

8   Begin just below the inguinal nodes in the groin. With one hand on the inner leg and the other on the outer side, cover as much of the circumference as possible; now squeeze inward and upward, 4 to 6 times.

9   Now place one hand on the front and one on the back and squeeze in an upward direction, 4 to 6 times.

10   Repeat this squeezing until the area softens.

11   As you feel the area softening slightly, perform small circular palmar kneading movements over the area (both palms pressing together). Cover the sides, front and back thoroughly.

12 Next, effleurage slowly towards the groin.

13 Move the hands down the leg, one hand width only at a time, overlapping the previous area. Repeat the manipulations as described. Work gently and slowly in this way until you reach the knee.

14 Now perform palmar kneading then effleurage over the entire thigh. As the tissues soften, deeper pressure may be applied and larger movements performed.

15 Move below the knee to drain the lower leg into the popliteal nodes. Begin just below the knee.

16 Avoid the anterior border of the tibia (shin bone). Cup the hands around the calf with the heels of the hands on either side of the shin bone. Squeeze in and upwards until the oedema softens. Vibrate the hands in and out. Knead the calf then effleurage.

17 Work gradually down the leg, one hand width at a time.

18 Work thoroughly around the ankles as fluid frequently stagnates around the medial and lateral malleoli.

19 Cup one hand behind the ankle joint – the thumb and thenar eminence on one side and the fingers on the other side of the Achilles' tendon. Place the other hand across the front of the joint.

20 Squeeze all the areas together in a pumping and upward push manner until the tissues soften. Work around the malleoli with the pads of the index, middle and ring fingers. Make small pressure circles around the bones. Then, with the fingers on either side of the Achilles' tendon, push in and up.

21 Press and knead the sole and dorsum of the foot with single-handed kneading.

22 Effleurage the lower leg again.

23 Effleurage the entire leg to complete the massage.

After the massage, active muscle contractions should be performed to exert a pumping action:

◎ pull foot up and down very slowly

◎ turn foot in and out

◎ circle foot around slowly

◎ tighten the quadriceps by pressing the back of the knee into the pillow and pulling the knee cap towards the groin

◎ repeat these movements 10–15 times.

Oedematous arm

The following routine is used to promote drainage of the upper arm into the axillary nodes:

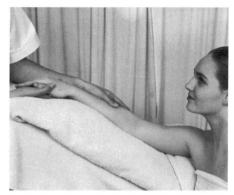

Figure 8.2 **Position of client with arm in elevation.**

| 1 | Elevate the arm to around 30°–45° or over – this is usually done with the client sitting on a chair, with the arm supported on a pillow on the elevated end of a plinth. Allow half to one hour for drainage. Make sure that the axillary nodes are neither stretched nor compressed. |

| 2 | Begin just below the axilla. Circle the arm with the hand – left hand underneath with fingers pointing medially, right hand over the top with fingers pointing laterally. Squeeze the tissues with inward and upward pressure. As the tissues soften, move the hands distally and overlap slightly. Repeat the squeezing down to the elbow. |

| 3 | Follow this with circular kneading over triceps and biceps. Place one hand on the triceps and the other on the biceps, then knead using small circles from the proximal to the distal end. |

| 4 | Effleurage the upper arm: begin proximally, push to axilla, return a hand width further down and push up again to axilla. Continue in this way until the hands reach the elbow. |

For drainage of the forearm, repeat the procedure, covering the area from the elbow to the wrist.

| 5 | Effleurage to the entire arm. |

Oedematous hand

| 1 | Place your left hand vertically behind the client's hand, and your right hand across the palm. Make small circular kneading movements with the palm into the client's palm. |

| 2 | Squeeze each finger and thumb gently. |

| 3 | Teach active movements of all joints of wrist, hand and elbow. |

❖ *Reducing cellulite* ❖

Cellulite is a condition, found predominantly in women, where areas of adipose tissue (fat) become hard and lumpy and very difficult to remove.

In women fat is found mainly on the outer thighs, hips and buttocks, abdomen, midriff and back of the arms. In men it is usually distributed around the waist. It is more common and more widely distributed in the female because of the greater amount of oestrogen produced. This hormone encourages the laying down of fat.

The areas of cellulite look dimpled or lumpy, and feel hard and cold to touch. Pushing the flesh between the hands makes the skin very uneven and puckered, similar to the surface of orange peel.

Cellulite is more commonly found in overweight individuals, but is also found in slim people and those of ideal weight. In the slim it is present in specific areas, usually the outer thighs, giving the characteristic 'jodhpur' shape. Cellulite is difficult to reduce and remove, even when the individual is on a reducing diet and exercising regularly. Research indicates that there is no physiological difference between cellulite and the more easily removed fat, but there are differences in the supporting connective tissue and in the organisation and circulation of the subcutaneous tissues in cellulitic areas.

The body stores fat for use as fuel when required. The digestive system breaks down the food we eat to provide energy for bodily functions. If the energy input is greater than the energy output (i.e. if we eat more food than is required for energy), then the excess fuel is stored in the body as fat.

Fat is stored in specialised cells called **adipocytes**. These form clusters supported by connective tissue, which group together to form adipose tissue. This is found under the skin in the subcutaneous layer, and among muscle fibres around organs such as the kidneys and heart. Complex chemical reactions convert the food eaten into fat for storage, and again from storage to use as fuel for energy. Although fat will be used from areas all over the body when required, it appears to be more difficult to remove from certain areas. These areas of hard, difficult-to-remove fat are called cellulite.

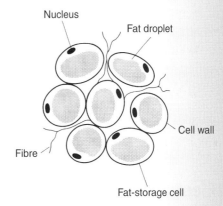

Figure 8.3 Storage of fat in adipocytes.

In cellulitic areas there is some alteration of the subcutaneous tissue. The adipocytes become overloaded and develop a tough outer membrane. The supporting connective tissue increases, enmeshing groups of adipocytes together in a lobular structure. This gives the dimpled, uneven appearance of the area.

The overloaded cells and lobules compress the capillary networks and lymphatics. This interferes with the circulation to the area. Stagnation and deficient circulation adversely affect the area: the tissues do not receive the required nutrients and oxygen; waste products (toxins) accumulate in the area as they are not quickly removed; and the temperature of the area will be lowered as warm blood is not circulating normally (hence it feels cold to touch). Fat remains in the overloaded adipocytes as it is not easily removed by the poorly circulating blood for conversion to energy, and the area becomes hard and stagnated. If action is not taken, the condition will become progressively worse, with greater engorgement of the area, degeneration of connective tissue and hardening of the fatty tissue.

Treatment techniques

The aims of the treatment are:

1 to soften and reduce the fatty adipose layer

2 to increase the circulation to the area, thus improving nutrition

3 to speed up blood and lymphatic drainage from the area, thus removing toxins more quickly

4 to improve the condition of the skin.

Successful treatment will involve combining a variety of treatments into an effective routine, which will include both manual and mechanical massage.

It is important to remember that spot reduction of fat from a specific area is not possible. To reduce body fat, calorie intake must be less than calorie output. Only then is fat removed from body stores and broken down for energy. The clients must therefore be given advice on sensible eating and made aware of the factors that are thought to contribute to cellulite (see 'advice to clients', on page 221).

A variety of treatments may be used to combat cellulite, but massage should always complete the treatment to improve drainage.

Electrical treatments

◎ **Electrical muscle stimulation** (EMS) to underlying muscles is effective because as the muscles contract and relax they exert a pumping action on the blood and lymphatic vessels. This stimulates the circulation in the deeper tissues and the metabolic rate of the area is improved. The sensory nerve endings in the skin will be stimulated and this will produce reflex dilation of the capillaries in the dermis, increasing blood flow to and from the area.

◎ **Galvanic treatment**, using the cathode over the area of cellulite, produces the alkali sodium hydroxide, which will soften the skin and tissues. It results in vasodilatation with hyperaemia and erythema, so more blood flows to and from the area. Water molecules are drawn towards the cathode, which will soften the area. Various anti-cellulite products containing negatively charged ions will be repelled by the cathode into the skin. These are designed to break down, and aid the dispersal of, cellulite.

◎ **Specialised body systems** using body wraps, clays, serums, creams and low-intensity currents are effective in stimulating the circulation.

◎ **Vacuum suction** is effective as it speeds up lymphatic and venous drainage of the area, removing fluid and toxins. Cups with reduced pressure are moved over the area in the direction of lymphatic drainage towards the nearest set of lymphatic nodes. The suction dilates the vessels as the cup moves along, increasing flow. Vacuum suction is effective after EMS and mechanical massage (G5). If combined with galvanic treatment it should be given first to decongest the area. *Do not use massage or vacuum suction after galvanic treatment as the areas under the pads are too sensitive*

◎ **Mechanical massage** (G5) produces a deeper effect and more stimulation of the body tissues than manual massage. The spiky head will stimulate and increase the circulation to the skin, producing an erythema. The increase in the delivery of nutrients and oxygen, the removal of waste products (metabolites), the increase in metabolic rate and the desquamating effect will all improve the condition of the skin. The deep kneading movements, using the 'eggbox' or hard spiked rubber heads, will affect the deeper tissues. The pressure of the strokes must be directed upwards to aid venous and lymphatic drainage. This massage warms and softens the area and speeds up the removal of metabolites. Heavy kneading movements should be brisk but not too prolonged, as resulting dilation of capillaries and blood vessels may increase the fluid in the area further, engorging it and increasing compression.

Manual massage

This forms an important part of the treatment and should conclude the treatment plan. As with mechanical massage, all manipulations must follow the direction of venous return and lymphatic drainage. As the flow in these vessels is speeded up, fluid and metabolites from tissue cells and spaces are removed more efficiently, reducing stagnation (stasis). The arterial circulation will in turn increase, bringing nutrients and oxygen to nourish the tissues, and the metabolic rate will increase. This improves the stagnant area. It may be that fat needed for fuel will be mobilised from this stimulated area, but there is no scientific research evidence to prove this.

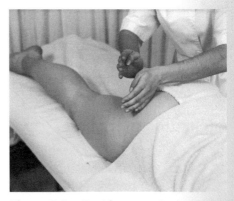

Figure 8.4   Hacking over the buttocks.

The heavier manipulations of kneading, picking up, wringing, hacking, cupping, beating and pounding may be used over the areas of cellulite, according to client needs. The greater the depth and the more consolidated and harder the cellulite, the deeper the manipulations should be unless the area is sensitive and painful, when manipulations must be within the tolerance of the client. Deep, brisk effleurage along the length of the area should conclude the massage.

If galvanic treatment has been used, remember that the area under the pads will be very sensitive. Therefore massage may be given proximal to (above) the area and around the padded areas to conclude the treatment.

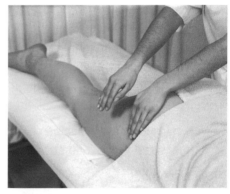

Figure 8.5   Cupping over the buttocks.

❖ *Male clients* ❖

The male client must be received with the same polite, caring manner as the female. As always, the highest standards of professionalism apply. Male and female therapists should avoid banter and ignore any suggestive comments or innuendo from clients of either sex.

Treatment technique
Preparation

1 Before the client undresses give clear instructions on use of the shower and covering towels, the return to the massage area and the positioning on the bed. Brief pants can be worn throughout the massage.

2 Position the towel widthways across the chest. Place a folded towel (double layer) across the lower abdomen. Place another towel lengthways over the previous towel and over the legs.

3 Men are frequently hairy and massage may be uncomfortable if insufficient oil or talcum powder is used. Talcum powder is often a better medium over hairy areas – apply liberally. If oil is used, ensure that it is not too viscous and again apply liberally.

Adaptation of strokes

1 Men generally have denser, firmer and larger muscles than women, depending on their degree of fitness. Massage manipulations may therefore be deeper and heavier, but this must be adapted to suit each client.

2 Stroking manipulations may be performed in the direction of hair growth, usually downwards. These movements should be light.

3 Effleurage should be performed in the direction of venous return, using plenty of oil or talcum powder. (If this pulls against the direction of hair growth or is uncomfortable, omit the movement.)

4 Petrissage manipulations also require care and a liberal amount of the massage medium.

5 More percussion manipulations may be included unless the client requires a relaxing massage.

6 Cover the body parts in the following order, omitting the abdomen:
  ◎ front of legs (avoiding the femoral triangle)
  ◎ arms – work over side of chest can be included with each arm
  ◎ back of legs
  ◎ back.

Where a male therapist is required to give massage to a female client, the chest and abdomen areas are omitted from the routine.

❖ *Evaluation of treatment* ❖

After each treatment it is important to assess how effective the treatment has been. You must decide whether the treatment has produced the effects that you were expecting, and whether the goals you set at the beginning have been met.

In order to evaluate the treatment you will need to obtain feedback: this means gathering all the information you can, which will indicate the effectiveness of the treatment. Knowledge of the results of the treatment will enable you to make changes or modifications next time should you feel that you have not achieved your goal.

You will obtain information through touch, i.e. sensing through your hands whether the tissues feel more flexible, pliable and less tense. You will also obtain information by looking at the area to see what changes have been produced. You will acquire more information through asking the client how s/he feels and whether the treatment met her/his needs.

As a result of the information you obtain from this feedback you will decide if changes need to be made and formulate a strategy for the next treatment. You have to make a judgement as to whether your selected treatment has been as effective as you hoped.

Through palpating the tissues you will sense whether the tissues feel more relaxed.

➤ Are the tissues softer?

➤ Are the tissues more flexible and extensible?

➤ Have fibrous or fatty nodules disappeared?

➤ Do the tissues feel warm but not too hot?

By looking at and examining the area you will obtain visual feedback.

➤ Is there a good even erythema?

➤ Are there uneven patches of erythema, which would suggest uneven pressure?

➤ Is the area very red and hot, which would indicate over-treating or a mild allergic reaction to the lubricant?

➤ Are there red sore spots over bony prominences indicating that these were not avoided?

By questioning the client you will obtain verbal feedback.

➤ How did that feel?

➤ Did you enjoy the massage?

➤ Did any part of the massage feel uncomfortable?

➤ Did it hurt anywhere?

➤ Was it as you expected it to be?

➤ Did you go to sleep?

➤ Was the pressure even throughout?

➤ Did you feel that you would have liked me to spend a longer time on any area?

➤ Was there any area that you would prefer me to leave out next time?

➤ Do you feel entirely satisfied with the treatment?

Allow the client time to relax and get up slowly. Discuss with the client any changes that you intend making next time and explain the reasons why they are needed. Record the results of the feedback and the strategy for following treatments on the record card. Always refer to these each time the client attends.

Give home advice as appropriate.

❖ *Home advice* ❖

Home care advice is very beneficial for the client, as it involves them in the treatment and encourages them to take control of their condition. It also provides linkage between one treatment and the next. The advice given will obviously depend on the client's need and condition, e.g. the overweight client or a client with cellulite will need dietary advice. For the tense, overworked client you may suggest that s/he tries to reduce her/his workload, that s/he makes time to rest, takes a relaxing bath and goes to bed early.

You may also teach relaxation techniques and advise her/him to practise these at home. Those with poor posture can be taught corrective exercises. Deep breathing exercises are helpful to everyone as they increase the intake of oxygen and the elimination of carbon dioxide. These techniques are explained in the following text.

❖ *Diet* ❖

Advice to clients

It is important that clients are made aware of the factors that are thought to contribute to the build up of fat and cellulite. They should be encouraged to follow a self-help, daily regime that will increase the efficiency of the treatment. The following home advice should be given:

1 Eat a well-balanced diet:
- ◎ include all the nutrients necessary for health, i.e. a little fat, proteins, carbohydrates, vitamins, minerals, water and fibre
- ◎ eat plenty of fresh fruit and vegetables (5 portions a day are recommended); do not overcook vegetables
- ◎ eat oily fish such as herring, trout, mackerel and salmon 3 times per week
- ◎ eat wholemeal foods such as wholemeal bread, pasta, rice, cereals, pulses, beans, nuts and seeds
- ◎ reduce intake of saturated fat found in butter, dairy products and red meat
- ◎ reduce intake of sugar and salt
- ◎ reduce intake of alcohol – 7 to 14 units per week only
- ◎ drink around 3 litres of water per day.

2 Balance energy intake with energy output:
- ◎ if the diet provides just enough energy to meet body requirements, there is no surplus to be stored, therefore no fat to be deposited. To reduce fatty tissue, energy input must be less than energy output. Only then will fat be utilised from body stores to provide required fuel

◎ reducing the diet and increasing aerobic activity is the best regime for reducing fat (e.g. walking, jogging, swimming or cycling for 20–30 minutes, twice to three times per week, is excellent).

3 Avoid wearing tight clothes that apply pressure and restrict the circulation, such as tight jeans or trousers, tight belts, underwear and corsets.

4 Take plenty of exercise and keep mobile during the day. If in a sedentary occupation, it is advisable to walk around, swing the legs and stretch at regular intervals.

5 Breathe correctly and deeply:
◎ practise deep breathing, thus using all areas of the lungs. Breathe in deeply and feel the sternum move forwards, the ribs move outwards and the diaphragm move downwards, pushing the abdomen out. Breathe out and feel the sternum move back, the ribs move in and down and the abdomen pull in
◎ when sitting or lying, breathing is shallow and uses mainly the upper chest. Deep breathing uses the chest capacity to the full and increases the intake of oxygen. The alternating pressure in the thoracic and abdominal cavities also stimulates the circulation around the body.

6 Eat plenty of roughage and drink 2–3 litres of water per day. This will aid digestion, prevent constipation and facilitate the elimination of waste products from the body.

❖ *Relaxation* ❖

Relaxation means being free from tension and anxiety, which are normally caused by the stresses of life, which upset the body balance. It is impossible to remove all the stressors in life and a certain amount of stress is desirable as it can produce feelings of thrill and excitement. The ability to relax is extremely important as it combats stress and reduces its harmful effects such as fatigue, lethargy, illness and psychological problems. Clients who lead very busy lives or are coping with worries or dealing with unhappy situations may find it very difficult to relax. Advising them and showing them ways of reducing stress and promoting relaxation can form an important part of treatment. Once they have recognised the difference between the tense state and the relaxed state they can continue to practise at home.

Preparation

The first consideration is to prepare the room or cubicle and create the right conditions to promote the relaxation response. These will be the same conditions required as those for massage treatment, namely:

➙ a warm, well-ventilated area

➙ a quiet area, away from distracting noise

- low and diffused lighting
- a spotlessly clean environment
- soothing décor in pastel colours
- a comfortable couch or mattress on the floor
- clean linen and towels for every client; these to be boil-washed after each use
- light blankets for additional warmth
- very soft, slow-moving music may be played if the client dislikes absolute quiet.

Relaxation techniques

There are many techniques that may be used to encourage the client to relax. They may be combined for maximum effect.

The relaxation response involves the client's response to a quiet soothing environment: total concentration on a particular object while trying to let go of all tension. This is sometimes sufficient to promote the relaxed state and can be practised anywhere.

Visualisation or imagining involves visualising pleasantly soothing situations conducive to relaxation, e.g. lying on a beach, looking at a tranquil scene etc.

Progressive relaxation aims to develop an awareness of the difference between feelings of tension and relaxation. Contraction followed by relaxation of all the muscle groups is performed, working around the body. This is a very effective method of promoting relaxation.

Progressive relaxation technique

Select and prepare a suitable area and prepare the client (see Chapter 3).

The client should lie on a mattress and be fully supported. The client may choose to lie on the back, in the recovery position or half lying if the client has difficulty in lying flat. The client must be well supported using plenty of pillows under the head, knees or as required. Allow the client a short time to settle and let go of tension. During this time encourage her/him to breathe deeply and let go as s/he breathes out.

The technique is then practised as follows, beginning with the feet and repeating each movement three times:

- Pull the feet up hard (dorsi-flexion), and let go
- Push the feet down hard (plantar flexion), and let go
- Push the knees down hard against the floor, and let go
- Push the leg down hard against the floor, and let go
- Tighten the buttock muscles hard, and let go
- Pull the abdominal muscles in hard, and let go

◎ Raise the shoulders, and let go

◎ Press the shoulders into the floor, and let go

◎ Press the arms into the floor, and let go

◎ Curl the fingers to make a fist, and let go

◎ Press the head into the floor, and let go

◎ Screw up and tighten the face, and let go

◎ Tighten all the groups together, and let go

◎ The client should breathe out on the 'let go'.

Use your voice to encourage relaxation when teaching these movements. The command 'tighten hard' can be used after each instruction with a firm voice, while 'let go' should be spoken in a lower tone and drawn out to encourage the feeling of letting go. The terms 'relax' or 'release' may be used in place of 'let go'.

The clients should be left to repeat the sequence on their own until they feel free of tension and sleepy. They may be allowed to sleep, time permitting, and woken up slowly. This sequence can be practised at home in a quiet place; it is particularly effective after taking a warm bath.

❖ *Posture* ❖

During the consultation the client's posture should be assessed. If there are postural problems then some muscles will be shortened and tight, while others will be stretched and weakened. These factors will influence the types of massage manipulation used over certain muscles. Tight shortened muscles will benefit from those manipulations that have a stretching effect such as the petrissage movements, while the stretched muscles will benefit from the more stimulating percussion movements.

Clients with poor posture will also benefit from exercises to correct posture; these can be given after treatment or as part of home advice.

Posture is used to describe the alignment of the body, in other words how the body is held. Very few people have perfect posture because it is influenced by both physical and psychological factors throughout life.

When the client comes into the salon, observe how s/he walks, stands and holds her/himself: this alone will give some information regarding posture. Are the movements evenly balanced or is there tilting, stooping or unevenness in the way s/he moves?

When the client has undressed, a more accurate assessment can be made.

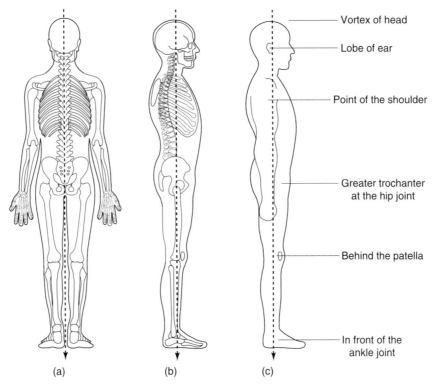

Figure 8.6   Points that the line of gravity will pass through if posture is correct.

Examination

Ask the client to adopt a normal stance and assess the posture from the front, side and back. A plumb line may be used to check body alignment: this should pass centrally down the front and back but at the side it should pass through the lobe of the ear, the point of the shoulder, the greater trochanter at the hip joint, behind the patella and in front of the ankle joint.

From the front

Head position:

◎   Are the ear lobes level? If they are not there is a muscle imbalance. The sterno-cleido-mastoid and the upper fibres of the trapezius are tight on the lower side, while those on the other side will be stretched.

Shoulders:

◎   Are they level, or is one higher than the other, indicating muscle imbalance? The upper fibres of the trapezius and levator scapulae are tight on the raised side. A difference in level may also indicate scoliosis, so check for that also. (A slight difference is considered normal.)

◎ Are both shoulders held high? This indicates tension in the muscles on both sides. The right and left upper fibres of the trapezius and the levator scapulae are tight.

◎ Are the shoulders drawn forward, rounded? This indicates muscle imbalance. The pectoral muscles are tight, but the middle fibres of the trapezius and rhomboids are stretched.

◎ Are there hollows above the clavicles? This indicates muscle tension, which may be due to respiratory problems such as asthma.

Breasts:

◎ Are the breasts held high or sagging? If there is breast sag and round shoulders, correction of the posture may help to lift the breasts.

Waist:

◎ Are the waist angles on the right and left level? If one is lower than the other, there may be spinal deformity or a difference in leg length.

Anterior superior iliac spines:

◎ Are they level? If not, there may be spinal deformity or a difference in leg length.

◎ Are they dropped forward? This indicates a lordosis with a tight erector spinae and quadratus laborum and stretched, weak abdominals.

◎ Are they dropped backwards? This indicates a flat back or sway back, with weak back extensors, i.e. the erector spinae and quadratus lumborum and tight abdominals.

Patellae:

◎ Do they point forwards? If not, there may be knock knees (genu valgum) or bow legs (genu varum).

Toes:

◎ Do they point forwards? If they point outwards there may be flattening of the medial arch and flat feet.

◎ If they point inwards or outwards, the weight distribution over the foot will be wrong, causing foot problems.

◎ Look for bunions, where the big toe deviates towards and sometimes lies across the other toes and there is swelling at the metatarso-phalangeal joint.

◎ Look for hammer toes, where the inter-phalangeal joints are deformed.

From the side

Use a plumb line. This should fall through the lobe of the ear, the point of the shoulder and the hip joint, behind the patella and just in front of the lateral malleolus.

Head position:

◎ Is the neck or cervical curve exaggerated and the chin forward? This means that the neck extensors, the upper fibres of the trapezius at the back of the neck, are tight and the neck flexors are weak.

Thoracic curve:

◎ Is there kyphosis, i.e. an exaggerated thoracic curve, giving a humped look? If so, the pectoral muscles are tight and the middle fibres of the trapezius and rhomboids weak.

Abdomen:

◎ Is the abdomen protruding or sagging forwards, indicating weakness of the abdominal muscles? The pelvis may be tilted forward. This is known as visceroptosis, as the weak abdominals allow the viscera to sag forward.

Lumbar curve:

◎ Is there lordosis, i.e. an exaggerated lumbar curve with the spine curved inwards? This means that there will be an anterior pelvic tilt with weak abdominals and tight erector spinae and quadratus laborum.

◎ If the lumbar region is flat, which is much less common, the erector spinae and quadratus lumborum will be weak.

Buttocks:

◎ Are the buttocks well toned with strong muscles, or are the gluteal muscles weak and sagging?

Knees:

◎ Are the knees hyper-extended?

From the back

Head:

◎ Are the ear lobes level or is the head tilted, indicating muscle imbalance? (see front)

Shoulders:

◎ Are they level? (see front)

◎ Are there winged scapulae, i.e. the inferior angle and medial border of the scapulae lift away from the chest wall? This indicates a weakness of the serratus anterior and the lower fibres of the trapezius.

Spine:

◎ Is there scoliosis, i.e. a lateral deviation of the spine? This may be an **S** or **C** curve to the right or left. If you are unsure, pull a finger down the spinous process: the red line should be straight, and will show up any deviation. A scoliosis may be structural (present from birth), or it may be postural, and will straighten out when the body is flexed forward.

Buttocks:

◎ Are the buttock folds level? If they are not, scoliosis, lateral pelvic tilt or different leg length may be present.

Heels:

◎ Are these square and firmly planted on the ground? If not, the weight distribution will be uneven.

Correction of the posture

The correction of the posture should begin at the feet. Each position should be maintained as the subsequent one is practised.

Feet

Stand with the feet 10 to 15 centimetres apart, with the toes pointing forward. The weight should be evenly distributed between the balls of the feet and the heels.

Practise the following:

◎ Raise the toes off the ground, feel the weight evenly distributed between the balls of the feet and the heels. Then lower the toes.

◎ Sway the body forward, feeling more weight on the balls of the feet.

◎ Sway the body backwards, feeling more weight on the heels.

◎ Position the body so that the weight is evenly distributed between the balls of the feet and the heels. Lift the medial arch slightly, but do not curl the toes.

Knees

◎ Press the knees backwards hard, ease the knees by bending them slightly, then find the mid-point and pull the kneecaps upwards by tightening the quadriceps muscle.

◎ If the knees are hyper-extended, ease them slightly and pull the kneecaps upwards as just shown.

◎ If the knees are bowed or knock-kneed, tighten the kneecaps, rotate the thighs outwards and tighten the buttocks to bring the kneecaps to point forward. Check the feet again after performing these movements.

Pelvis

◎ Tilt the pelvis forwards and then backwards; pull it forwards again tightly, tucking the tail under, and hold this balance. Pull the abdomen in and breathe out as the pelvis is pulled forward, then hold this position while breathing normally.

Thorax

◎ Pull the thorax upward from the waist as you breathe in, drawing the shoulders backwards and downwards. Hold this position while breathing normally. Do not thrust the chest forwards.

Neck and head

◎ Elongate the neck and pull the chin backwards. Feel as though someone is pulling the hair upwards at the crown.

Check the feet, knees, pelvis and thorax again, hold this position and then relax. Practise this correction several times a day and during various activities; correct the posture during inhalation and hold the balance during exhalation.

If the new posture is maintained while walking around, it will eventually become habitual.

Home practice of posture correction

You must ensure that the client is always aware of the difference between good and poor posture. Poor posture may be the result of long-term habits. These habits must be changed through constant practice of correct positions.

Explain this to the client and give simple pointers, which s/he must practise as often as possible. Good posture will become automatic through constant practice.

➤ Look straight ahead with the eyes level.

➤ Pull the chin in, then relax into a neutral position (neither pulled in nor craned forward).

➤ Feel that the crown of the head is being pulled up towards the ceiling.

➤ Keep the neck straight but not tense.

➤ Pull the shoulders back and down; do not hold the chest forward.

➤ Hold the tummy in and tuck the tail under.

➤ Balance your weight evenly through the buttocks if sitting, or through the feet when standing.

Common postural problems and corrective exercises

Kyphosis

This is an exaggerated curve of the thoracic region.

The weak stretched muscles that require strengthening are:
the middle fibres of trapezius, the rhomboids and the middle part of erector spinae.

The tight muscles that require stretching are:
pectoralis major and the neck extensors.

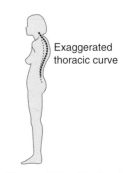

Exaggerated thoracic curve

Figure 8.7   Kyphosis.

CORRECTIVE EXERCISES

Sitting or stride standing – gently drop the head forward pulling chin in, press the head back making a long neck and raise.

Lax stoop sitting – raise the trunk gradually from the base of spine upwards.

Lying, arms at right angles with elbows bent – retract the shoulders pressing back of hand into the floor.

Prone lying, hands clasped behind back – keep chin in, pull shoulders back and lift head and shoulders off the floor.

Lordosis

This is an exaggerated curve of the lumbar spine where the pelvis is tilted forwards.

The weak stretched muscles that require strengthening are:
the abdominals – rectus abdominus, internal oblique and external oblique
the hip extensors – gluteus maximus and the hamstrings.

The tight muscles that require stretching are:
the trunk extensors – erector spinae and quadratus lumborum
the hip flexors – ilio-psoas.

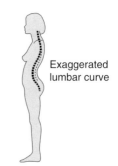

Exaggerated lumbar curve

CORRECTIVE EXERCISES

Crook lying – press small of back into the floor and pull tummy in, tilting the pelvis.

Figure 8.8   Lordosis.

Crook lying – keep chin in and raise head and shoulders to look at the knees; progress to curl up.

Prone kneeling – arch the back to stretch the lumbar spine and return to horizontal.

Prone kneeling – keep the back straight, raise alternate legs out and up; keep knee bent.

Scoliosis

This is a lateral curvature of the spine, which may be a long **C** curve or an **S** curve.

The muscles that will require strengthening will be those on the outside of the curve. The muscles that require stretching will be those on the inside of the curve.

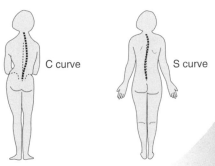

Figure 8.9   Scoliosis.

CORRECTIVE EXERCISES

Stride standing – reach up into the air with the arm on the concave side of the curve; reach towards the floor with the other hand. Stretch, hold, relax.

Stride standing – side flex the trunk towards the convex side, where the muscles are stretched. Slide the hand down the side and return.

Prone lying – stretch the arm on the concave side up above the head along the floor; stretch the other down towards the feet. Hold and relax.

Prone lying – stretch the arm on the concave side up above the head and the opposite leg down along the floor. Hold and relax.

Flat back

This is a condition where there is little or no lumbar curve and the pelvis is tilted backwards. It may be accompanied by kyphosis of the thoracic spine.

The weak stretched muscles that require strengthening are: the back extensors, namely erector spinae (in some cases the abdominals and gluteus maximus are weak).

The tight muscles that require stretching are: the hamstrings on the posterior thigh.

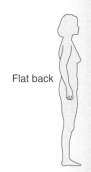

Figure 8.10   Flat back.

231

CORRECTIVE EXERCISES

Sitting – lean forward, taking the pressure from the buttocks on to the thigh, then extend the back to create a lumbar lordosis. Hold for a count of ten then release.

Prone lying – raise alternate legs.

Prone lying – raise both legs (this exercise is allowed for this condition).

Prone kneeling – arch and hollow the back.

Long sitting – rotate the pelvis forward, then lean backwards to arch lower back.

❖ *Breathing exercises* ❖

Breathing exercises are given to maintain and improve the expansion of the chest. This increases the amount of oxygen taken into the lungs and increases the amount of carbon dioxide out of the lungs. Breathing in is known as *inspiration*, and breathing out is known as *expiration*. As explained in Chapter 2 the muscles of respiration are the external intercostal muscles and the internal intercostal muscles (which lie between the ribs) and the diaphragm, which lies horizontally separating the thoracic cavity from the abdominal cavity. The contraction of these muscles will increase the capacity of the thorax from side to side, from front to back and longitudinally from top to bottom.

Effects of breathing exercises

- improve the mobility of the thorax
- increase the intake of the oxygen, which will improve metabolism
- increase the output of carbon dioxide thus eliminating this waste product more quickly
- improve the condition of the lungs
- loosening lung secretions
- the changing pressure created in the thorax aids the flow of blood in the veins and the flow of lymph in the lymphatic vessels
- the increased mobility of the thorax improves posture.

Technique

Position sitting on a chair or lying. Remove any tight restricting clothing.

Deep breathing concentrates on three areas of expansion, namely, apical, costal and diaphragmatic.

Apical breathing; place the hands on the upper chest below the clavicle, breathe in deeply through the nose and expand the chest under the hands. The chest will move up and forward as you breathe in; then breathe out through the mouth and the chest will move back as you breathe out. Try not to allow movement in the other parts of the chest. Repeat 3 times.

Costal breathing; place the hands on the side of the ribs, above the waist. Breathe in deeply through the nose and feel the ribs moving out sideways; breathe out through the mouth and the ribs will move back as you breathe out. Repeat 3 times.

Diaphragmatic breathing; place the hands in front, above the waist. Breathe in deeply through the nose and feel the lower chest and abdomen moving forward as you breathe in; breathe out through the mouth and pull the abdomen back in as you breathe out. Repeat 3 times.

Then breathe deeply using all areas of the chest as follows: breathe in deeply through the nose, hold to count of 5 and breathe out for as long as possible through the mouth. Repeat 3 times.

Practise yourself before teaching clients to ensure that you fully understand the movements. Deep breathing can make one feel dizzy and faint because the amount of oxygen and carbon dioxide in the body is changing and the balance between these chemicals is disturbed. If this occurs then it is important to rest for a few minutes until the feeling passes and the balance is restored. This must be explained to clients before they are encouraged to practise at home.

❖ *Evaluation of own performance* ❖

To judge how you have performed, ask yourself the following questions:

◎ Did I make sure that everything was in place prior to the client's arrival? i.e. the room (to ensure a suitable, quiet environment), the couch (clean linen, towels and pillows), the trolley (neatly laid out with all commodities to hand).

◎ Did I abide by the salon's health, safety and hygiene policies?

◎ Did I adopt a friendly, relaxed, professional, competent manner?

◎ Did I respect the client's privacy and dignity?

◎ Did I observe the client's body language?

◎ Did I adapt my approach to suit the type of client?

◎ Did I make the client feel at ease?

◎ Did I communicate well with the client; was I polite, sensitive and supportive?

◎ Did I carry out a detailed client consultation and record the information on a treatment card and get it signed by the client?

◎ Did I note all contra-indications and take the required action?

◎ Did I allow the client the opportunity and time to express her/his needs and expectations?

◎ Did I listen closely to what s/he was saying?

◎ Did I select the most suitable treatment and set long-term goals?

◎ Did I explain everything clearly to the client and did s/he understand my explanation?

◎ Did I agree the treatment plan, cost and timing with the client and obtain her/his written consent?

◎ Did I maintain eye contact with the client?

◎ Was I aware of my own body language?

◎ Did I make the client feel secure, comfortable and cared for?

◎ Did I select the best possible treatment to suit the client?

◎ Did I select the most suitable lubricant and make sure I did not waste any?

◎ Did I wash my hands before treatment?

◎ Did I adopt the correct posture and position to avoid strain, injury and fatigue?

◎ Did I use a variety of suitable manipulations at the correct pressure and rhythm?

◎ Did I check the well-being of the client during the treatment?

◎ Did I evaluate the treatment outcomes?

◎ Did I offer home advice?

◎ Did I keep within the time constraints for a viable cost-effective treatment?

◎ Did I dispose of all waste into a lined bin with a lid?

◎ Did I clean the treatment area and leave it tidy?

This list will also help you to prepare for a massage assessment, as it demonstrates pointers to successful performance.

QUESTIONS

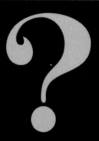

1. List six conditions or problems that will benefit from massage.
2. Explain why it is important for the treatment room to be warm, well ventilated and quiet.
3. Give three important considerations of technique when giving massage for relaxation.
4. Explain what is meant by the following:
   (a) visual feedback
   (b) verbal feedback.
5. List six reasons why clients may feel tired and lethargic.
6. Give two manipulations that may be used for invigorating a tired client that would not be used in a relaxing massage.
7. Explain why the part should be elevated when giving massage to relieve oedema.
8. Explain why movements for relieving oedema should begin proximally and not distally as in a general massage.
9. Give the three main movements used when treating oedema.
10. Describe the appearance of cellulite.
11. Give two areas of the body where cellulite is found in women.
12. Give four aims of treatment when dealing with cellulite.
13. List two other treatments that may be used in conjunction with massage for the treatment of cellulite.
14. Explain why care must be taken when using massage following galvanic treatments.
15. Explain briefly the home advice you would give a client who wished to reduce areas of cellulite.
16. Explain how you would adapt the massage for a male client.

9 Additional techniques

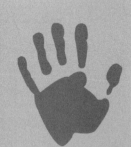
❖ *Massage techniques for musculo-skeletal problems* ❖

Clients requesting massage frequently complain of pain or stiffness in localised areas of the body, most commonly in the back muscles and the posterior muscles of the neck. Problems may be identified during assessment or when the hands move over the part during a general body massage: these will require further investigation. When the area is palpated, changes may be detected in the tissues that indicate underlying abnormalities of the skin, connective tissue and underlying muscles.

236

The following changes may be found:

- → Muscles may feel hard and tight, indicating increased tension or shortening.

- → Tissues may feel thick and unyielding with little or no pliability or flexibility.

- → Areas may be tender, painful or hypersensitive to touch, indicating neural (nerve) involvement.

- → Fibrous bands, nodules or points of extreme irritability (trigger points) may be felt as the hands move over the part.

A general massage will promote relaxation of these tissues, but deeper and more specific techniques are required to identify the problems and bring about improvement.

The individual components of the musculo-skeletal system must function normally in order to produce full-range, pain-free movement, and any problems or changes in one part will affect the others.

The tissues involved will include:
the muscles (muscular), which produce movement; the bones onto which the muscles attach, and the joints where movement occurs (skeletal); the connective tissue (fascia), which connects and separates other tissues; the blood and lymphatic vessels of the area, which deliver nutrients and oxygen and remove the waste products of metabolism (metabolites); and also the nerves (neuro), that is, the sensory nerves that transmit sensory stimuli to the brain, and motor nerves that transmit impulses from the brain to the muscles to initiate movement and control tension. Under normal stress-free conditions the CNS maintains a level of muscle tone that allows normal pain-free movement. Abnormalities such as adhesions entrap nerves and disturb the normal neurological activity between the central nervous system and the musculo-skeletal system, which will affect muscle tone and normal function.

Stress in any one part of the system will affect all the other adjacent parts as they are all interdependent. Neuromuscular techniques aim to normalise the tissues and restore normal neurological control.

Causes of musculo-skeletal problems

There are many factors that contribute to problems of the musculo-skeletal system.

The more common causes are:

Trauma and injury

Injury will result in pain and damage to the joints, bones, muscles, ligaments, tendons or nerves. The extent of the damage and the degree of pain will depend on the severity of the injury. The trauma may result in:

- ➤ strains of muscles or tendons, where the fibres may be overstretched or torn

- ➤ sprains of the ligaments that support joints, which may tear or rupture

- ➤ extreme forces dislocating joints and/or fracturing bones

- ➤ tears or disruption of the connective tissue layers

- ➤ increased pressure or damage to nerves

- ➤ damage to blood vessels and lymphatic vessels resulting in bleeding and fluid seeping into the tissues, resulting in swelling of the area

- ➤ a protective spasm of the surrounding muscles as the body attempts to prevent further movement, thus limiting and containing the damage. This is an automatic response controlled by the central nervous system.

The area may be hot, red and swollen, and there may be pain on movement, with loss of function. The heat and redness are due to dilation of the blood vessels, while the swelling is due to fluid seeping out of the blood vessels into the tissues: this is known as exudate. This fluid exudate contains cells and plasma proteins, in particular fibrinogen, which forms fine threads of fibrin. As healing progresses, some of the fluid is reabsorbed but some remains in the tissues together with the fibrin threads. This exudate thickens further and the fibres are laid down in a haphazard manner, forming cross-bridges within the tissues.

This binds the tissues together forming thickenings, tight bands and nodules. The increased tension and pressure will irritate the nerve endings resulting in areas of tenderness and pain.

The healing of wounds involves the formation of fibrous scar tissue, which contracts and hardens over time. The amount of scar tissue formed will depend on the size of the wound. Scars and fibrous adhesions bind tissue fibres and layers together, preventing smooth movement, and glide over one another. The tissues lose flexibility and extensibility both lengthways and widthways, and the range of movement is limited. Appropriate massage manipulations can help to loosen these adhesions, realign the tissue fibres and restore their extensibility and pliability thus increasing the range of movement, relieving pain and restoring full function.

Massage must be avoided in the acute stage of injury and the initial stages of healing as it may cause further damage. It should only be considered when healing is complete.

Postural problems

Posture is the term used to describe the alignment of the body. Good posture means that the body is balanced and the muscle work required to maintain it is minimal. Poor posture means that the body is out of balance and certain muscles must contract strongly to maintain the position. Habitual, long-term poor posture will result in some muscles over-contracting and shortening while their antagonists (opposite group) lengthen and weaken.

Posture is influenced by many factors, such as a sedentary life style, taking little exercise, poor working conditions, or poor sitting or working postures such as sitting and looking at a computer screen all day, with shoulders rounded and the head craned forward. Back and neck problems are often the result of poor posture.

It is thought that the muscles that maintain the shortened position actually tighten and shorten and their connective tissue becomes tighter and less flexible. The increased tension in these contracted muscles impedes the circulation, resulting in a decrease in the delivery of nutrients and oxygen and a build up of metabolites (waste products of metabolism). This results in stiffness, pain and greater tension.

Nodules and thickened areas may develop in these muscles as a few fibres exhibit extreme tension. The causes of postural problems will need to be identified and rectified through exercise and improved postural habits.

Massage will help by promoting relaxation of the tightened muscles. In addition, stretching techniques and flexibility exercises may be used to restore length to shortened muscle fibres, and mobility to connective tissue.

Strain as a result of repetitive movements (RSI)

Individuals who perform repetitive movements over a long period of time may be over-loading and over-using their muscles. Tendons and their sheaths may become inflamed, producing pain on movement. Some muscles may be constantly working in shortened positions, resulting in increased tension and adaptive shortening. Joints may be forced to the extreme end of their range. This will alter the stresses and forces on the supporting ligaments and on connective tissue, which contracts and tightens. The circulation will be restricted resulting in fatigue, pain and stiffness.

The cause of the problem must obviously be identified, rectified and eliminated if possible. Specific massage techniques are used to stretch connective tissue and free ligaments and tendons around the affected joints. Flexibility exercises and stretching techniques are also given to increase joint movement and aid full function.

Tension produced by psychological or emotional factors

Certain psychological and emotional states can produce increased tension in the muscles. Fear, anxiety and stress can cause the muscles to be held in a rigid state, which produces tenderness and pain. Introverts and those who are sad, upset or timid will exhibit poor posture resulting in problems already described. Tension exhibited over a period of time may result in adaptive shortening of the tissues, restricted circulation and increased pressure on nerve endings, resulting in pain and stiffness.

General body massage will help to relieve general stress but specific techniques are required to improve areas of extreme tension and to elongate the tissues.

Chilling of the tissues

Cold will increase tension in the tissues, the muscles contract, and the circulation is restricted. Low temperature will also cause vasoconstriction, which further reduces the blood supply. If the chilling is of short duration then the tissues recover quickly but some stiffness will remain. Longer-term cooling, such as sitting in a draught for a period of time, can decrease the pliability of connective tissue, resulting in pain and stiffness. Massage is used to aid relaxation of the tissues, to produce vasodilation and increase the blood flow to the area. This increased blood flow, together with the heat produced through hand contact with the part, will warm the area, increasing the pliability of the tissues. Stretch techniques are used to improve flexibility and extensibility of the tissues.

Disease of the joints

The most common diseases are inflammatory and degenerative arthritis, but there are many others that cause primary changes in the joints and secondary changes to the surrounding soft tissues.

Massage must not be given in the acute stages of joint disease, when the joint may be red, hot, swollen and very painful.

During the chronic stage when pain has subsided, gentle massage may be used to soothe and relax the tissues, and aid the absorption of any swelling. When the disease has completely 'burnt out', localised massage techniques performed around the joints will help to reduce swelling, and loosen the ligaments and tendons. This may be followed by gentle passive and active movements.

Palpation of the tissues

When abnormalities are present in the tissues, they are detected through the palms of the hands or the pads of the fingers, as these have large numbers of sensory receptors. This probing and feeling for changes and abnormalities is known as palpating the tissues. The ability to palpate the tissue layers accurately and identify abnormalities is extremely important because selection of the appropriate treatment is based on these findings. This skill requires a lot of practice and a great deal of experience.

Problems may be identified during consultation; during a general massage while performing effleurage or stroking movements; or during specific exploratory movements. Palpation is best carried out on dry skin without any lubricant, although this is not always possible, as a lubricant may have already been applied before the problem was identified. It is then better to continue the massage and return to the localised area towards the end, when the lubricant will have been absorbed. Palpation is mostly done with the pads of the fingers or thumb, as these are the more sensitive areas of the hand, but sometimes the whole palm is involved, 'feeling and sensing' the tissues as it moves along. Pressure is adjusted depending on the depth of the tissue being palpated. Light pressure is required for palpating the skin and superficial fascia, becoming heavier for muscle and bone.

Remember that you are looking for abnormalities: explore the tissues under the hand and feel for thickened areas or nodules. Then move the tissues around, and sense the pliability and stretch in the tissues. Note anything that feels different from the surrounding areas, and compare it with the other side for guidance. Are there areas of tenderness or pain that produce a reaction from the client? When conditions are identified then appropriate techniques can be selected to improve and normalise the tissues.

Abnormalities

Any of the following abnormalities may be encountered as you palpate the tissues:

Pain

Contact with the part may elicit pain: it is important to obtain verbal and non-verbal responses. The client will be able to describe the pain but always be aware of the client's reaction when and as you touch her/him. If you can see her/his face, does s/he grimace with pain? If s/he is lying prone and you cannot see her/his face, watch for body reaction. If s/he is feeling discomfort or pain s/he will twitch and move away from your touch. Ask her/him to describe the pain: is it sharp or dull? How severe is it? On a scale of 1–10 when 1 equals no pain and 10 equals intense pain, where does her/his pain lie?

Pain is a symptom of some underlying cause or stress: when pain is present the underlying cause must be identified. Pain may be *acute*, that is, sharp and of sudden onset, indicating the acute stages of injury or disease, when massage is contra-indicated; or pain may be *chronic*, that is, deep, dull pain, which may be the symptom of a long-standing chronic condition. The pain may come on gradually and develop slowly; it may be fairly static or may steadily increase; or it may be intermittent or constant and difficult to relieve. It may radiate over a large area or it may be localised to small points within muscles or fascia, which may be extremely painful when touched.

Intractable pain must always be medically investigated, that is, any pain whether it be dull, throbbing, sharp, severe etc, which never diminishes nor is relieved by rest. There may be a serious underlying cause, and massage should not be carried out.

Pain is not always felt in the immediate vicinity of the problem: it may radiate away from the exact site. It may be referred to another area some distance away that has the same nerve supply, e.g. tension in the neck muscles can refer pain to the head. Malfunction of internal organs can refer pain and produce changes in superficial tissues that share the same nerve root, e.g. problems in the liver may refer pain to the skin area below the right scapula.

Muscle tension

A mild degree of tension is present in healthy skeletal muscle at all times and is known as muscle tone. It ensures that the muscle can contract quickly in response to a stimulus. This tension may increase in response to many factors such as pain, injury, postural or psychological problems, as previously outlined. As tension increases, pain increases due to pressure on and reflex activity of the nerves. More pain results in greater tension, setting up a tension/pain cycle.

Increased *tension* produces *pain*, which results in *further tension*, which produces more *pain*.

Tension over a period of time will result in physiological changes within the tissues. There will be circulatory changes, due to increased pressure on the blood vessels. The blood supply to the area will be limited, oxygen and nutrient supply will be reduced, and metabolites will build up. At this stage there will be aching and soreness in the muscles, and they will feel hard and unyielding when palpated. If tension is prolonged the muscles and fascia will shorten and contract and will feel tight and rigid.

This will result in loss of elasticity and flexibility: the muscles resist sideways movement and efforts to lift them from underlying structures. All these factors limit function and produce further pain.

General massage routines will help to relieve tension and improve the circulation but localised and more specific techniques will be required if the pain is chronic, with thickened hypersensitive areas in the tissues.

Oedema

This is swelling of the tissues, which can often be seen without the need to palpate. The skin and underlying tissues will appear tight with loss of pliability.

Any swollen area should be palpated very gently, as the skin will be stretched and may break down easily. If it is not too severe, the swelling will feel soft and spongy while severe swelling will feel hard and unyielding. Chronic oedema of long standing feels dense and firm to touch: *pitting* will occur when pressed with the thumb, i.e. the indentation made by the thumb will remain in the flesh for some time but will eventually refill with fluid.

The build up of fluid will increase the pressure within the tissues, which presses on the nerves and stimulates the pain receptors, resulting in pain.

Massage can aid the removal of fluid from the tissues but it is very important to establish the cause of the oedema, as massage does not help all cases. Treatment of oedema is explained on pages 210ff.

Fibrous adhesions

As explained previously, the healing processes following injury or inflammation may result in the fluid exudate and fibrin forming fibrous adhesions among the tissues. These are laid down in a haphazard manner and limit the flexibility and extensibility of the area. Adhesions may form within the muscles following micro tears of the fibres, or they may develop within the superficial and deep layers of fascia as a result of stress or trauma. They may also form around ligaments and tendons, binding them down to underlying bone. Adhesions form cross-bridges or bonds within the tissues, preventing the smooth glide of the tissues over each other during movement. They restrict the lengthening and sideways movement of the fibres. The tissues feel dense, stiff and less pliable and movement is limited in all directions.

Fibrous adhesions within a muscle or in the connective tissue layers surrounding the muscle will restrict the elasticity and full lengthening of the muscles. This will limit full-range movement and may produce pain on movement.

Massage manipulations such as stroking and myofascial release techniques are used to stretch the fibrous adhesions in all directions and also to realign them. Flexibility and extensibility are increased, and normal movement of the tissues is restored.

Fibrotic nodules

These are hardened, lumpy zones usually painful to touch, lying within superficial muscles or fascia. They are small areas of tense contracted fibres with restricted circulation. The tight, hardened nodule may be mobile, that is, it moves within the tissues when gently pushed around; or it may adhere to the underlying tissues when there is little movement. They tend to be painful in the area of the nodule but do not refer pain to other areas. Nodules are treated with pressure techniques: the degree of pressure used is dictated by the amount of pain produced, which must be within the tolerance of the client. Pressure may be increased as the pain subsides. Nodules frequently disappear when the pressure is applied.

Fatty nodules

These are lumps of fatty tissue within the fascia: they feel softer than fibrous nodules and can be moved around more easily. They are usually less painful and disperse more easily with pressure. They are treated with pressure techniques.

Trigger points

These are small areas of hypersensitive contracted tissue. They may produce pain over the exact location of the trigger point, which may radiate over the surrounding area, or the pain may be referred to another area known as the target zone. The pain in these areas increases with pressure. They are treated with pressure techniques: see further for a full explanation.

Crepitus

This sounds and feels like fine crackling among the tissues. It results from inflammatory changes within the tissues. When acute inflammation subsides, it may leave a chronic thickening and dryness in the tissues.

❖ *Neuromuscular-skeletal techniques* ❖

These techniques should not be viewed as apart from general massage movements, but rather as additional skills that may be used to relieve pain and restore function to localised conditions. They may be incorporated into a general body massage or may form part of the routine for a specific part of the body, such as the neck or back. Localised tissue abnormalities may be identified during consultation or during the course of a body massage. The appropriate techniques must then be selected and extra time spent on these areas to bring about improvement.

These techniques are sometimes referred to as bodywork techniques, soft tissue manipulation, neuromuscular treatments etc. They all use pressure and/or stretch manipulations to reduce tension, ease pain and stiffness, and to restore full function. Specific manipulations are used to target the following conditions: increased tension within muscles (hypertension): thickening or fibrous adhesions within the tissues (muscles or connective tissue); contracted fascia; small areas of hypersensitive tissue (known as trigger points); fibrotic or fatty nodules.

The techniques included in this text are neuromuscular stroking technique; myofascial stretch/release techniques; trigger point therapy. Deep effleurage and frictions can also be used, as explained in Chapters 4 and 5 respectively.

The therapist must adopt a sensitive, caring and gentle approach, bearing in mind that these manipulations are aimed at releasing abnormal tension within the muscles. Through reducing and normalising neural (nerve) activity, relieving hypersensitive areas, stretching contracted tissue, realigning fibres, and restoring flexibility and pliability to the tissues, the continuing cycle of pain–tension–more pain is interrupted and normal function is restored. Contra-indications are the same as those for general massage.

Neuromuscular stroking

This involves sensitively searching through the tissues for abnormalities such as areas of increased tension, dense thickened areas, loss of pliability, and manipulating them. The area is explored in all directions using stroking movements with the thumb or fingers. Superficial pressure is used for assessing and treating superficial tissues but deeper pressure is required for assessing and treating the deeper tissues.

Anatomical knowledge of the area is essential, in particular, knowledge of muscle shape and fibre direction. If you are unsure, refer to a muscle chart or detailed diagram before commencing the treatment. This is extremely important because, as you palpate through the area, some strokes are performed across the fibres to loosen adhesions and reduce thickenings but other strokes are performed along the fibres to release tension and realign the fibres.

The *aims* of this treatment are to release areas of hypertension and contracted tissue; to loosen adhesions and realign tissue fibres; to increase the pliability of thickened tissue; and to reduce pain and restore normal function.

Uses

◎ to identify abnormalities in the tissues

◎ to stretch contracted thickened tissue

◎ to realign tissue fibres

◎ to reduce reflex activity through the nervous system

◎ to reduce tension

◎ to relieve pain

◎ to restore full function.

Effects

Superficial manipulations will produce the following effects:

◎ the skin and superficial fascia are loosened and mobilised

◎ the elasticity of the skin and superficial fascia is improved

◎ adhesions are stretched and loosened thus improving the glide between the superficial and deep fascial layers

◎ the circulation of blood and lymph is increased to the superficial tissues, improving their condition.

Deeper manipulations will produce the following effects:

◎ stretching of the deep fascia will improve its flexibility

◎ when the fascia is stretched and separated, the glide and movement between the deep fascial layers, and between the fascia and the muscles, is improved, thus smooth movement of the tissues is facilitated. Mobility increases and the tension decreases

◎ the movement and the heat generated by the hand on the part increases the pliability of the fascia

◎ stretching and softening of any fibrotic adhesions within muscles or fascia will reduce tissue tension and restore flexibility

◎ the tissue fibres that have become distorted by stress or the pull of adhesions are realigned along their normal lines of stress. Muscles are then more able to withstand sudden stresses applied to them. This will limit damage such as micro tears of the fibres

◎ decreased tension within the muscles reduces the pressure on sensory nerve endings, thus reducing pain

◎ the pressure manipulations and relaxation of the tissues decrease neural reflex activity, hence the pain cycle is interrupted

◎ blood and lymph are able to circulate more freely through the tissues, therefore the delivery of oxygen and nutrients is increased and the removal of irritating chemical metabolites is speeded up. The physiological functioning of the whole area improves.

Treatment technique

To palpate the tissues, move the pads of the fingers or thumb superficially over the tissues and search carefully for any areas that feel harder and less pliable than normal. These will be areas of increased tension, thickening, fibrotic adhesions or nodules. Continue moving deeper into the tissues with increased pressure to locate the exact site of the problem. When abnormalities are identified, the area should first of all be warmed with general manipulations such as effleurage and kneading and then treated with the deeper stroking movements. The treatment is completed with more effleurage.

Strokes may be long or short, depending on the size of the area. Short strokes are used for small areas of tension but longer strokes are used on larger areas. Strokes may be applied with the fingers, the thumb, and sometimes with the elbow when deeper pressure is required.

When the thumb is used contact is made with the lateral border of the ball of the thumb while the fingers rest lightly on the part. For greater pressure, both thumbs may be used, positioned one behind the other with the fingers of both hands resting on the part. Alternatively, the pads of the fingers may be used: on small areas contact is made with

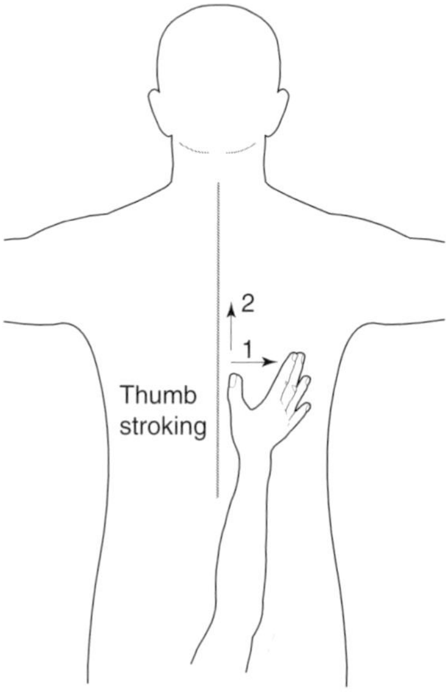

Figure 9.1 Neuromuscular stroking on erector spinae.

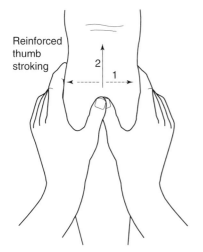

Figure 9.2   Neuromuscular stroking on gastrocnemius.

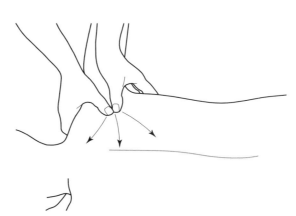

Figure 9.3   Neuromuscular stroking to trapezius and the rhomboids.

the middle finger supported by the index and ring fingers but on larger areas the three fingers may make contact reinforced by the same fingers of the other hand.

Stroke over the area in all directions to stretch the tissues and loosen any adhesions. Then stroke in the direction of the muscle fibres until the tissues yield or give slightly: this will elongate and realign the tissues. Repeat several times until any pain is reduced and the area feels softer and more pliable. Effleurage the area to complete the treatment. This stroking technique can also be used to treat fibrotic and fatty nodules.

Trigger point pressure

Trigger points are small, hard areas of extreme irritability, usually located within a muscle but can also be found in the fascia. They are tender and painful: the degree of pain can vary from mild discomfort to excruciating pain. When palpated they feel like short, thick, tight bands of contracted fibres, which produce a 'twitch' when stroked. The muscles in which trigger points are located may be tense and shortened, their elasticity is limited and they are unable to extend to their normal length. Pain is usually produced when the muscles contract or are stretched or manipulated.

Trigger points may be described as *latent* or *active.*

Latent trigger points are painful only when direct pressure is applied.

Active trigger points are tender, radiate pain, and may also refer pain to another area known as the target zone, or target area. This occurs because the trigger point and the target zone are innervated by the same spinal nerve or are linked by the autonomic system.

Trigger points develop in muscles and fascia following trauma or when extreme tension develops and the tissues are held in a shortened position over a period of time. This increased tension increases pressure on nerve endings resulting in pain and also restricts the blood circulating through the area. The supply of nutrients and oxygen is reduced, metabolites, including chemical irritants, build up in the muscle and the normal physiological functioning of the area is disturbed. The chemicals irritate the sensory receptors in the tissues, resulting in more pain.

IDENTIFYING TRIGGER POINTS

Trigger points may be found as the hands move over the part during a general massage or during palpation to identify the cause of pain or tenderness in an area.

The pads of the fingers are more sensitive at detecting changes in the tissues but the whole palm may also be used. Light to moderate pressure is applied depending on the degree of pain. The hands move very slowly and gently over the area until a very tender spot is encountered. The client may seem anxious and twitchy, may attempt to move away from your touch, or may even cry out in pain.

The following *signs* will indicate the presence of a trigger point:

➤ Pain is produced or increased in the exact location of the trigger point when pressure is applied and/or pain may be referred in the target zone.

➤ A tight rope-like band can be felt in the tissues.

➤ A twitch response occurs when the finger slides over the area.

➤ The client describes the pain as extremely tender and attempts to move away from the pressure.

Uses of pressure techniques and stretching

◎ to deactivate the trigger point and relieve pain

◎ to relieve the tightness/spasm of the muscle fibres

◎ to improve the circulation and return normal physiological function

◎ to stretch the muscles and return to full-range movement.

Effects of pressure techniques and stretching on trigger points

◎ The initial pressure applied will increase the pain but as the pressure is maintained or increased, the pain will decrease. This is due to factors that reduce the activity of the nervous system, i.e. the nervous system adapts to the pressure, and sensitivity of nerve endings is reduced; the chemical metabolites that irritate the nerve endings are reduced; and the release of endorphins (the body's natural analgesic), which suppress pain, is possible.

◎ When pressure is applied into the trigger point, the underlying blood vessels are compressed and the blood is squeezed out; when the pressure is released, the blood vessels dilate and fill with fresh blood. This alternate pressure and release continually flushes the area with fresh blood, which will remove the build up of metabolites including chemical irritants, and also bring oxygen and nutrients to the tissues thus aiding return to normal physiological function.

◎ As pain is relieved during the treatment then the degree of tension in the muscle decreases because it breaks the pain cycle (pain–tension–pain).

◎ The stretching techniques that are applied after the pressure treatment also reduce spasm in the muscle fibres. In addition they loosen and realign the fibres, which improves extensibility and lengthening of the muscle.

Treatment technique

In an attempt to deactivate a trigger point, direct pressure is applied at 90° to the fibres. Pressure can be applied through the pads of the thumb or fingers, or through the elbow. As the pressure is applied it must activate the trigger point: consequently the pain may initially increase. The client may feel the pain at the exact point of pressure only, or the pain may also be referred to a target zone but it should be just bearable for the client. If the pressure is too great, it will make the client tense up: this is obviously counter-productive. If the trigger point is extremely sensitive, treatment should commence with light pressure, deepening as pain diminishes, but it must always be within client tolerance.

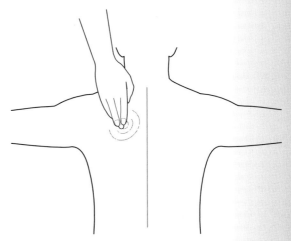

Figure 9.4   Finger pressure to trigger point at medial border of scapula.

The pressure is maintained for approximately 6–12 seconds until the pain diminishes, the pressure is then released, and after a few seconds is reapplied until the tension in the tissue eases and the pain subsides. The client should be instructed and encouraged to relax into the pain. This helps to break the pain–tension cycle. If the pain continues to increase and does not ease, release the pressure and stop the treatment as there may be an underlying inflammatory condition that is a contra-indication.

Following the direct pressure technique, the shortened muscles should be stretched (using the stretch techniques already described) and every attempt made to restore elasticity and full length.

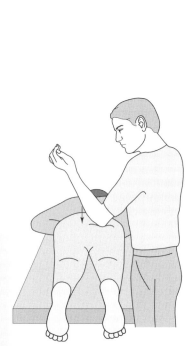

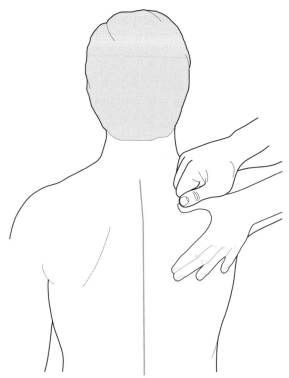

Figure 9.5 Elbow pressure to trigger point in gluteal muscles.

Figure 9.6 Thumb pressure to trigger point in trapezius.

Myofascial-release manipulations

These techniques work on the muscles and the fascial layers of the body. Fascia is areolar tissue: it is an irregular connective tissue composed of a loose arrangement of collagen and elastin fibres in a viscous ground substance. It is the most widespread tissue in the body: it connects and supports tissues and organs.

It is laid down in large sheets throughout the body, connecting skin to muscle; wrapping around muscle bundles; connecting muscles to each other and to bone; and is found supporting organs and lining body cavities. There are three types, located in different areas of the body.

Subcutaneous fascia, which lies beneath the skin and is a continuous layer all over the body. It connects the skin to the underlying tissues and in the normal state allows smooth movement between the two.

Deep fascia, which lies in sheets and bands around and between muscles. It binds muscle fibres into bundles, and muscle bundles together; it surrounds the entire muscle and also lies in layers between muscles, linking them together and attaching them to the bones. Pliability and flexibility of this deep fascia is therefore essential to facilitate smooth movement during contraction and relaxation of the muscle. When conditions are normal the connective tissue is pliable and allows full movement of the muscle but under abnormal conditions, when the fascia becomes thickened, tight and inflexible, full-range movement will be limited.

Subserous fascia, which lies between the deep fascia and the serous membrane that lines the body cavities. It supports organs and facilitates movement between them (these techniques will not reach or affect this layer).

Connective tissue is capable of change: it becomes more pliable with movement and temperature increases, but becomes tight and inflexible with tension and cold. Following trauma or when abnormal postures are held over a period of time, the connective tissue in the area thickens and becomes more fibrous. It becomes less pliable and may cause distortion of the tissues. These sheets of fascia interconnect throughout the body and any tightness or distortion in one area may cause problems in another.

Any of the pre-mentioned causes can result in tightening of the connective tissue with distortion and limited function of adjacent tissues, e.g. injury, postural or psychological problems.

The *aim* of myofascial techniques is to realign fibres, to soften and increase the mobility and pliability of the fascia and restore full function.

Identifying myofascial problems

The skin and the superficial tissues will feel less mobile. There will be a general thickening and loss of pliability in the area. The movement of the skin over the underlying tissues will be restricted and the tissues feel less flexible. The client may complain of stiffness or/and a dull ache.

Assessment of the posture will indicate any areas held in shortened positions, e.g. a forward-poking chin will result in shortened cervical tissues and posterior neck muscles. Lordosis will result in shortening of the tissues and muscles of the lumbar region.

Uses

◎   to restore mobility to the fascia

◎   to release the subcutaneous layer from the skin

◎   to release deep fascia from the muscle

◎   to soften thickened fibrous areas

◎   to restore pliability and flexibility

◎   to correct any distortion of the tissues

◎   to restore normal movement and function

◎   to relieve stiffness and pain.

Effects of myofascial techniques

◎ The skin and superficial fascia are lifted away from the underlying tissues: this loosens and improves the flexibility of the skin and fascia.

◎ The deeper techniques stretch the deep fascia, realign the collagen fibres and release any cross-bridges.

◎ Flexibility of the fascia is improved, therefore adjacent muscles are able to function normally.

◎ The circulation to the area is increased, partly due to the alternate pressure and release on the vessels, but also because the tightness between the fascial layers, which restricts blood and lymphatic circulation to the tissues, is released. When fascial tension is released, blood and lymph flow improve, and tissue fluid passes more freely through the fascia. The tissues receive more nutrients and oxygen, and the rate of removal of waste products is increased, therefore condition and function of the tissues improve.

◎ When tension in the tissues is released, extensibility improves, which aids the return to full function.

Myofascial treatment techniques

These techniques are used to stretch the tissues: the first two techniques stretch the skin and superficial fascia while three and four are aimed at the deeper fascial layers. These techniques are applied without any lubricant because the skin must not slide under the hands.

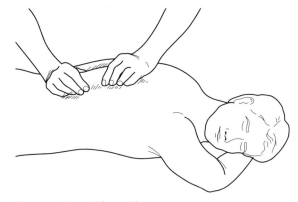

Figure 9.7   Skin rolling.

1   *Skin rolling* may be used to release superficial fascia, and is frequently performed on the back, over the ribs. Place the hands on the part with the thumb abducted, lift and push the flesh with the fingers towards the thumbs, and roll this flesh with the thumbs, back towards the fingers. Repeat 3–4 times as needed, then move on to an adjacent area.

2   *Vertical lifting technique* may be used to lift the skin and superficial fascia away

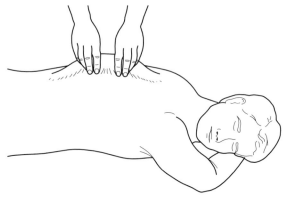

Figure 9.8   Vertical lifting technique.

from underlying tissues. The hands are positioned vertically above the part, and fingers and thumb are held straight and pointing towards the tissues. The skin and superficial fascia are grasped between the fingers and thumb, and lifted directly upwards, held for a few seconds and then released. This is repeated 3–4 times in one area and then the hands move along to the adjacent area. Take care not to pinch the flesh; the effort is directed towards the lift.

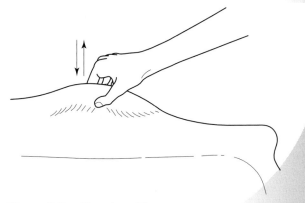

Figure 9.9 Muscle rolling.

3   *Muscle rolling technique*, this is usually used on the long-limb muscles. Place the muscles in their shortened relaxed position. Grasp the muscle between the fingers and thumb; the larger muscles will fill the palm. Lift the muscle if possible, then push it away from you and then pull towards you. Pull and push the muscle transversely in this way several times, to stretch and release the fascia. On long muscles it will be necessary to move along the muscle, and repeat the lift and pull/push again.

4   *Stretch–release* is a technique that targets the muscles and deeper fascial layers. The stretch must be applied in the direction of the muscle fibres. It is performed slowly and requires great concentration and ability to feel the resistance, and then the yield, in the tissue. With the arms crossed, one hand anchors the skin while the other hand applies movement in the opposite direction, pushing the skin and fascia horizontally until the point of resistance is felt. This point is held until the tissues release and yield slightly. Repeat the stretch until there is no further release. The hand then moves on to another area. Take care not to slip and chafe the skin.

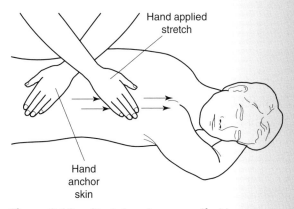

Figure 9.10   Stretch–release applied by one hand.

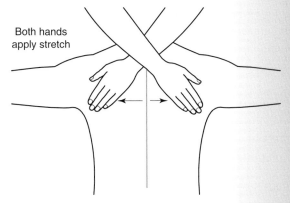

Figure 9.11   Stretch–release applied by both hands.

A similar *stretch–release* technique involves placing the crossed hands on the skin and moving them apart. Pressure is applied through the ulnar border of the hands as they move away from each other. Stretch is applied to the underlying tissues, held for a few seconds at the end of the stroke and then released.

❖ *Passive movements* ❖

Passive movements may be incorporated into massage routines to aid client relaxation. The therapist carefully moves the client's joints through as full a range as possible. Normally the movements we perform are the result of muscle contraction. Muscles contract in response to impulses/stimuli from the brain and spinal cord transmitted via motor nerves to the muscles. As the muscles contract, they pull on the bones at the point of attachment, and movement occurs at the joints over which they pass. This is known as **active** movement.

Movement at joints can also be produced by an external force, such as another person moving the joint when the muscles are relaxed, that is, not contracting.

This is known as **passive** movement.

DEFINITION

Active movement is controlled by the nervous system, which stimulates the muscles to contract and produce movement at the joints. It may be *voluntary* movement, which is under the conscious control of the client, such as moving the arm; or *involuntary*, which is not willed by the client but is a reflex movement such as blinking.

Passive movement is performed by an external force while the muscles are relaxed, usually one person moving another person's joints.

There are three grades of passive movements, namely *relaxed*, *forced* and *manipulative*, depending on the degree of force used.

This text relates to **relaxed passive movements** because both forced and manipulative movements are medical procedures.

(If movement is limited by adhesions or contractures, forced passive movements are performed to move a joint just beyond its existing range, while manipulative passive movements aim to return the joint to full-range movement. Greater force is required in the manipulative procedures and the person is sedated.)

Relaxed passive movements are movements performed by the therapist while the client's own muscles are relaxed. The joints are moved through the existing range: that means the fullest range possible without applying force.

(The range of movement may be restricted if the joint has been affected by disease or damaged through injury in the past. Any damage or erosion of the bone surfaces or residual adhesions will produce tightness and eventually contractures of the soft tissues around the joint, which will limit the movement.)

It is very important to assess accurately the possible range at each joint and work to this limit, offering only slight overpressure.

If the disease or injury is acute then passive movements are contra-indicated.

Joint structure

The classification, structure and factors that affect the range of movement of joints are explained earlier (see Chapter 2). You must revise and understand these facts before performing passive movements. The different types of synovial joint have different movements.

Relaxed passive movements are performed on synovial joints, which are the moveable joints of the body. For full range of movement to occur, e.g. from full extension to full flexion, all the component structures of the joint must function normally. During acute injury or disease, passive movements must not be carried out: following recovery there may be residual problems that affect the movements at the joint and the therapist must be aware of these.

Study the parts of a synovial joint: it will help you to understand the following:

Common conditions that affect joints

Two common conditions that affect the structure and function of joints are rheumatoid arthritis and osteoarthritis. Although differing in pathology, they both result in damage to the hyaline cartilage that lines the bones, inflammation of the synovial membrane and an increase in synovial fluid entering the joint space. These factors produce heat, swelling and pain around the joint, which limit movement.

Inflammation may spread to other structures surrounding the joint such as the capsule, ligaments and tendons. The inflammatory exudate (fluid) tends to thicken and solidify, forming adhesions among the tissues. At the same time, the muscles around the joint will contract and shorten in response to pain (this is the body's protective mechanism to resist movement, thus protecting the body from further pain).

Injuries and other conditions involving the joint may also result in degeneration, adhesions and shortening of the soft tissues (i.e. the capsule, ligaments, tendons and muscles around the joint). These factors will result in stiffness, tightness and contractures, which will limit the range of movement.

Changes and shortening of the soft tissues initially produce tightness of the joint, which can be rectified by giving passive movements and flexibility exercises. However, if no treatment is given, the tissues will continue to shorten and become bound down resulting in fixed permanent contractures.

Tightness will limit the movement but can be rectified and a return to full-range movement is possible, but when *contractures* develop the problem can only be rectified by forced passive movements or surgical manipulative procedures.

Consultation

Passive movements are usually integrated into a massage treatment, therefore a full client consultation and assessment will have been carried out. During the consultation it is important to ask specific questions relating to joints.

- ➤ Do you have any pain in any of your joints?

- ➤ Have you suffered from joint pain in the past?

- ➤ Have you ever injured any joints or fractured a bone near a joint?

- ➤ Do you suffer from stiffness in any joint?

- ➤ Have you had any bone- or joint-related illness, either lately or as a child?

- ➤ Do you ever have swelling of any joints?

- ➤ Have you noticed any bony growths around any joint (will indicate that changes have taken place in the joint, produced by arthritis or past trauma)?

Positive answers to any one of these questions will mean that great care must be taken during treatment or may mean, if the condition is severe, that treatment must not be carried out.

Contra-indications to passive movements

Examine the joints carefully and ask appropriate questions. If any of the following conditions are present then the treatment should not be carried out.

Bone fractures: avoid working on the affected limb until healing is complete; the other unaffected limbs can be treated.

Swelling of the joint: swelling may indicate some damage to the joint and passive movements are contra-indicated. However, if there is no damage, swelling around the ankles may be due to an accumulation of tissue fluid: passive movements combined with massage can then be carried out to improve this condition.

Hot or painful joints: these signs indicate that pathological changes are occurring in the joint.

Recent or active arthritic conditions: the joint will usually be hot, stiff and swollen.

Open wounds, cuts and abrasions near the joint: risk of increasing the bleeding; risk of infection and blood contamination.

Bruising around the joint: risk of further bleeding; healing must be complete before commencing treatment.

Recent sprains of the joint: healing must be complete before commencing treatment.

Recent strains of any muscle around the joint: healing must be complete before commencing treatment.

Recent scar tissue: there is a danger of breaking down scar tissue. However, when the scar is completely healed (after about six months) passive movements may help to stretch it.

Dysfunction or disorders of the nervous system: such as multiple sclerosis, strokes, Parkinson's disease etc. These conditions should be treated by therapists specialising in this field.

Spasticity in the muscles, i.e. muscles with increased tone: pulling against spastic muscles may increase the spasticity.

Metal pins or plates within a joint or within the bones forming the joint: these will have been inserted to stabilise the joint or bone following trauma. There is the risk of displacing or loosening these pins.

Thrombosis or phlebitis: these conditions are explained in Chapter 3. Although the muscles are not actively contracting during passive movements, the alternate stretch and release of the muscles acting on the joint may be sufficient to dislodge a blood clot from the vein wall, releasing it into the blood stream. The clot may then be carried to a vital organ such as the lungs where it may cause a blockage of the blood supply with potentially fatal consequences.

Skin infections and very fragile skin: there is a risk of spreading an infection and also of cross-infection. If the skin is very thin and fragile, great care must be taken to avoid splitting or causing open sores.

Uses of passive movements

◎ to maintain and slightly improve the existing range of movement

◎ to prevent the formation of adhesions

◎ to prevent stiffness of the joint

◎ to aid relaxation.

Passive movements in a massage routine should move each joint smoothly and rhythmically through all its movements. The client is relaxed and *neither* assists nor resists the movement. Passive movements will have an effect on all the structures inside and outside the joint.

Effects of passive movements

Passive movements will:

◎ maintain the present range of movement. Moving the joint as far as possible each time and giving slight overpressure will ensure that the range is maintained

◎ prevent tightness or stiffness of the joints

◎ maintain the extensibility of the soft tissues around the joint

◎ prevent the formation of adhesions

◎ stimulate the production of synovial fluid and lubrication of the joint

◎ may slightly assist venous and lymphatic flow as the muscles are stretched and relaxed over the moving joint

◎ have a soothing and relaxing effect if done slowly and rhythmically.

Technique of passive movements

Ensure that you know the anatomy and direction of movement of each joint. Remember that the movements will be different depending on the type of joint. The hinge joints of the knee and elbow can move to flexion and extension only, while the ball and socket joints of the shoulder and hip can move through flexion, extension, abduction, adduction, medial and lateral rotation and circumduction.

Explain the procedure to the client; ask if s/he has any questions and encourage her/him to relax. If you are including passive movements in your massage routine do not interrupt the flow and continuity to explain the procedure, but include this in the initial explanation and discussion with the client.

Maintain the highest standard of client care and hygiene throughout.

Check that the client is comfortable and that all areas not being treated are covered and supported.

Adopt the correct stance and maintain good posture throughout. Stride standing is the most common position but some movements require a change to walk standing.

Fix the joint: movement should only occur at the joint being worked on. The joints above and below should be fixed. This is done either by your hand support or by positioning the limb on the plinth for support.

Grasp above and below the joint firmly but gently: pressure should be even and constant, do not pinch or dig in to the client, and avoid bony points.

Apply slight traction: when you have a firm hold on either end of the joint, apply a slight, gentle pull, giving traction to the joint surfaces.

Move the joint smoothly, slowly and rhythmically to the end of the range, giving slight overpressure, then move back in the opposite direction.

Complete the movements of one joint before moving smoothly on to the next.

Move each joint through the fullest range possible without applying any force.

Take care not to overstretch the structures supporting the joint as this could result in damage to the joint. It is quite easy to avoid this, because at the limit of each movement you will become aware of the 'soft end feel' of the movement. This is the point at which you apply very gentle pressure to gain a little extra movement. It takes a little practice to become aware of this point.

Consider the speed, which must be moderately slow, even and rhythmical. Remember that the aim is to relax the client.

The joints to be treated and the number of movements performed should be decided upon at commencement of the treatment and should be the same for each joint and for each side of the body. This will depend on the purpose of the treatment and the time constraints when these movements form only part of the whole treatment plan. Repeat the movements 4–6 times.

Passive movements to joints of the upper limb
With the client in supine lying.

If passive movements are used for relaxation only, it is usual to limit hand movements to flexion and extension or to omit them altogether and begin at the wrist joint. They are, however, included in this text for those who may require them for mobilisation treatments.

Hand
The *joints* are:

1 interphalangeal joints, i.e. joints of the fingers
movements: flexion, extension of the fingers

2 metacarpo-phalangeal joints, i.e. the knuckle joints
movements: flexion and extension, abduction, adduction.

Procedure for finger joints: Fix the client's hand by holding with one hand across the palm, at the base of the metacarpals. Place the other hand behind the client's hand along the fingers.

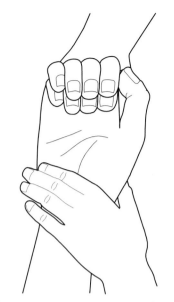

Figure 9.12   Flexion of the fingers.

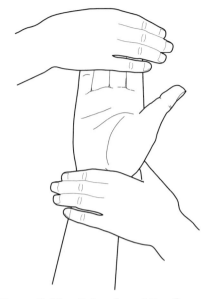

Figure 9.13   Extension of the fingers.

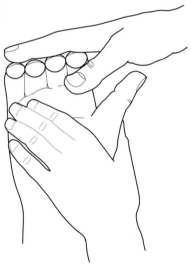

Figure 9.14   Flexion of the knuckle joints.

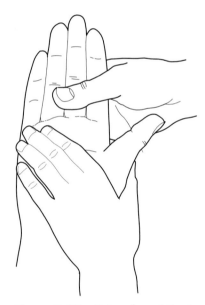

Figure 9.15   Extension of the knuckle joints.

Fully flex all the fingers together into the palm of her/his hand, then slip your hand up over the tips of her/his fingers and extend them.

Procedure for the knuckle joints: Fix the client's hand by holding low down the palm, level with the base of the thumb. Place your other hand behind and across the client's fingers with your thumb in front across the base of the fingers. Fully flex the knuckle joints then extend them.

The **thumb** can be omitted unless there is a particular reason for mobilisation.

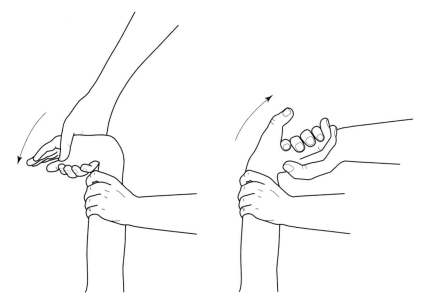

Figure 9.16   Flexion of the wrist.   Figure 9.17   Extension of the wrist.

The two interphalangeal joints should be individually flexed and extended by holding below and above the joint.

The *saddle joint* at the base of the thumb (near the wrist) has the following *movements*: flexion, extension, abduction, adduction, circumduction and opposition.

Place your hand across the wrist to fix it and use the other hand to move the thumb: take care not to overstretch as the saddle joint is susceptible to stiffness and pain.

Wrist joint

The *movements* are flexion, extension, abduction, adduction and circumduction.

Place one hand around the forearm about two inches proximal to the wrist, rest the upper arm on the bed and flex the elbow to 90°: fix in this position. Hold the client's hand firmly, with the other hand across the palm and move the wrist, first into flexion and extension; then into abduction and adduction; then circumduction.

Radio-ulnar joints (superior and inferior)

The movements are supination and pronation.

With the arm extended, hold firmly with one hand just above the elbow to fix it. The other hand holds the client's hand as for a hand shake. Keep the wrist in mid-position and turn the forearm into pronation and supination.

Elbow joint

The movements are flexion and extension.

With the client's arm resting along the bed, cup the elbow in your hand to fix the upper arm. Hold the client's wrist with your other hand preventing movement at this joint. Now flex the elbow until the flexor surfaces make contact preventing further movement. Then extend the elbow taking care not to hyperextend, i.e. extending beyond the normal limit. Use the hand that is cupped around the elbow to feel or sense the end of range and to give support at this point.

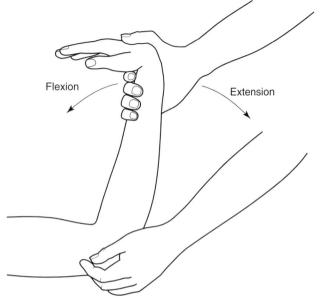

Figure 9.18   Flexion and extension of the elbow.

Shoulder joint

The movements are flexion, extension, abduction, adduction, medial rotation, lateral rotation and circumduction.

This is a complex ball and socket joint with many planes of movement. The arm can be taken through flexion into elevation, i.e. taken above the head. It may also be taken from abduction across the body into horizontal flexion. Perform these movements yourself until you are confident of each direction. When including passive movements for relaxation purposes it is easier to maintain rhythm and continuity by limiting shoulder movements to abduction, adduction, flexion/elevation and extension. However, for mobilisation all movements must be included.

PROCEDURE FOR ABDUCTION AND ADDUCTION

Hold the arm behind the elbow, with the other hand at the wrist; or place one hand over the shoulder to stabilise it, thumb in front and fingers behind. Grasp the client's upper arm just above the elbow allowing her/his forearm

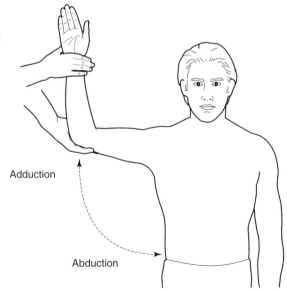

Figure 9.19   Abduction and adduction of the shoulder joint.

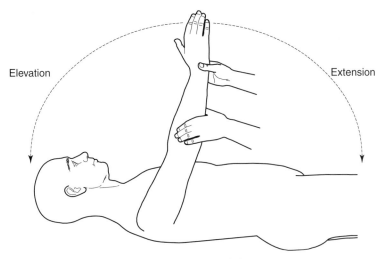

Figure 9.20   Elevation and extension of the shoulder joint.

and hand to rest across the therapist's forearm. Keep the arm level with the body and move it away from the body by 90° into abduction, then return it to the side of the body into adduction.

PROCEDURE FOR ELEVATION THROUGH FLEXION AND EXTENSION

Hold the client's arm just above the elbow and hold the wrist with the other hand; rotate the arm laterally and lift it upwards above the client's head, then bring it down into extension. This movement will be limited by the bed unless the client is lying along the edge of the bed. It is not desirable to move the client if these movements are part of a treatment when limited extension is acceptable, but the client should be moved if the purpose is mobilisation.

PROCEDURE FOR HORIZONTAL FLEXION AND EXTENSION

Hold the client's arm just above the elbow and hold the wrist with the other hand as shown. Abduct the arm to 90°, then take it across the body (at chest level) into flexion and bring it back as far as possible into extension (in the abducted position).

PROCEDURE FOR MEDIAL AND LATERAL ROTATION

Grasp the client's arm just above the elbow with one hand and hold the wrist with the other. The upper arm can rest on the bed. Take the client's arm into abduction, then rotate it backwards into lateral rotation and then forwards into medial rotation.

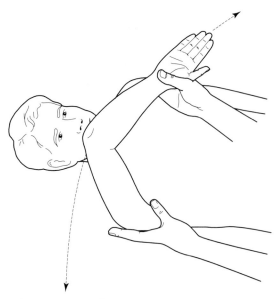

Figure 9.21   Horizontal flexion and extension.

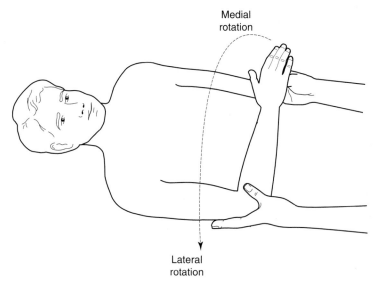

Figure 9.22   Medial and lateral rotation of the shoulder joint.

Passive movements to the joints of the lower limb

With the client in supine lying.

If passive movements are given for relaxation only, the toe joints can be omitted. However, these movements are important if the objective is to mobilise the joints because contractures and curling of the toes affect gait and can be very disabling.

Toe joints

1 Interphalangeal joints: movements are flexion and extension.

2 Metatarso-phalangeal joints: movements are flexion, extension, abduction, adduction.

Hold the foot firmly at the head of the metatarsal joints with one hand, place the other hand over the toes then flex and extend them all together or one at a time. Abduction and adduction is then performed individually at the metatarso-phalangeal joints. Pay particular care and attention to the big toe, as movement at this joint may be painful and restricted due to deformity and a bunion.

Ankle joint

The movements are plantar flexion (pointing the toes down) and dorsi flexion (pulling the foot up).

Place one hand behind the heel, cupping it in your palm. Grasp the foot firmly with the other hand around the metatarsals. Move the foot upwards into dorsi flexion and then downwards into plantar flexion. Ensure that you push beyond the 'soft end feel' of each movement especially dorsi flexion, as it is important to maintain the stretch on the Achilles tendon that passes down the back of the leg to insert into the calcaneum. Greater stretch of this tendon can be produced by holding the heel in the palm of your hand with the foot lying along your forearm. The other hand holds above the ankle and the foot is pushed up by the forearm into dorsi flexion.

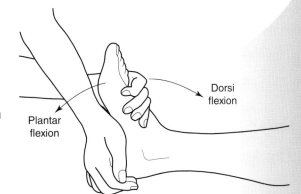

Figure 9.23 Dorsi flexion and plantar flexion of the ankle joint.

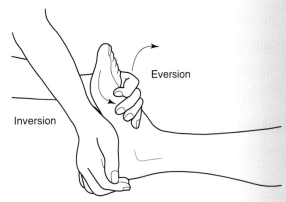

Figure 9.24 Inversion and eversion of the ankle joint.

The mid-tarsal joints

The movements are inversion and eversion.

Fix the ankle with one hand and hold the foot at the instep and turn it inwards and outwards. A combination of the movements just shown will produce circumduction, i.e. circling the foot.

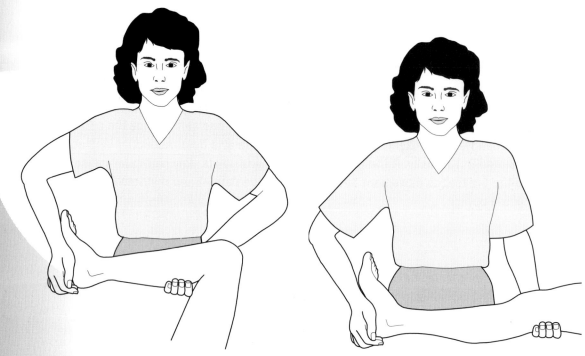

Figure 9.25 Flexion of the knee joint.   **Figure 9.26 Extension of the knee joint.**

The knee joint

The movements are flexion and extension.

Cup the heel in one hand and place the other hand behind the knee across the popliteal fossa. Give support with this hand to prevent the knee falling into hyperextension. Fully flex the knee and bring the hand from the back of the knee to the front just below the knee to give overpressure. This will also flex the hip joint. The knee is then moved into extension, sliding the hand back to the popliteal fossa for support and preventing hyperextension.

Flexion and extension of the knee can also be performed in the prone lying position with the foot over the edge of the bed. One hand is placed on the lower thigh while the other hand grasps above the ankle. The knee is then flexed and extended.

The hip joint

The movements are flexion, extension, abduction, adduction, medial and lateral rotation and circumduction.

PROCEDURE FOR FLEXION AND EXTENSION

Flexion of the hip joint will have been performed with flexion of the knee as already explained. Full extension of the hip joint can only be carried out in prone lying or side lying. In prone lying with the client's foot over the edge of the bed, place one hand on the buttock. The other hand is placed under and above the knee with the client's lower leg supported along the forearm.

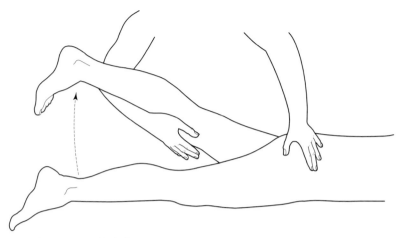

Figure 9.27   Extension of the hip joint.

Lift the straight leg into extension. Ensure that movement does not occur in the lumbar spine, by applying pressure downwards on the buttock and preventing the anterior aspect of the joint raising off the bed.

Both these movements can be carried out in side lying but the weight of the leg must be supported by the therapist, making the manoeuvre cumbersome and difficult.

PROCEDURE FOR ABDUCTION AND ADDUCTION

Place the leg not being worked on into abduction: support the moving leg by cupping under the ankle with one hand while the other hand supports under the knee preventing hyperextension. Keep the leg in line with the body and take it out sideways into abduction and back across mid-line into adduction.

PROCEDURE FOR MEDIAL (INTERNAL) AND LATERAL (EXTERNAL) ROTATION

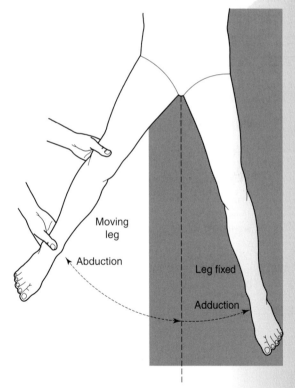

Moving leg

Abduction

Leg fixed

Adduction

Figure 9.28   Abduction and adduction of the hip joint.

With the legs slightly apart but supported on the bed throughout, place one hand on the thigh and the other on the lower leg. Grasp the leg gently and turn it inwards and outwards. For continuity it is suggested that hip joint flexion is carried out with knee joint flexion: this is then followed by abduction, adduction, medial and lateral rotation, with the client in the supine position. S/he is then asked to turn over into the prone position, and extension of the hip is carried out.

❖ *Body brushing* ❖

This treatment is used to improve the texture of dry, flaky, rough skin. It is usual to treat the entire surface of the body but it may also be used on legs and arms only. Manufacturers produce a range of different products and specific routines that may vary slightly from each other but the basic technique is the same for all. The following text will provide you with the basic technique, which can be adapted according to the specific requirements of your salon. Prepare the couch, and cover with a disposable paper sheet.

Effects

1 Desquamation, the removal of dead, flaky skin, improves the texture of the skin.

2 Surface capillaries dilate, increasing the blood supply to the skin and improving skin tone.

3 The increased blood supply will increase the metabolic rate of skin cells, which will improve the condition of the skin.

4 Lymphatic drainage is increased thus removing waste products and fluid from the tissues.

Precautions

➤ Check for contra-indications

➤ Ensure that the brush is securely held and strapped in your hand

➤ The pressure must be light and even over the parts

➤ The brush stroke must end at the nearest set of lymphatic nodes

➤ Follow each brush stroke with a hand stroke to maintain personal contact and to improve the comfort of the client. Brush with one hand, stroke with the other

➤ Cover each area well: three strokes on each part in the same order.

Treatment technique

Preparation of the client.

◎ Place the client in a well-supported comfortable position

◎ Check that all jewellery has been removed

◎ Explain the treatment to the client

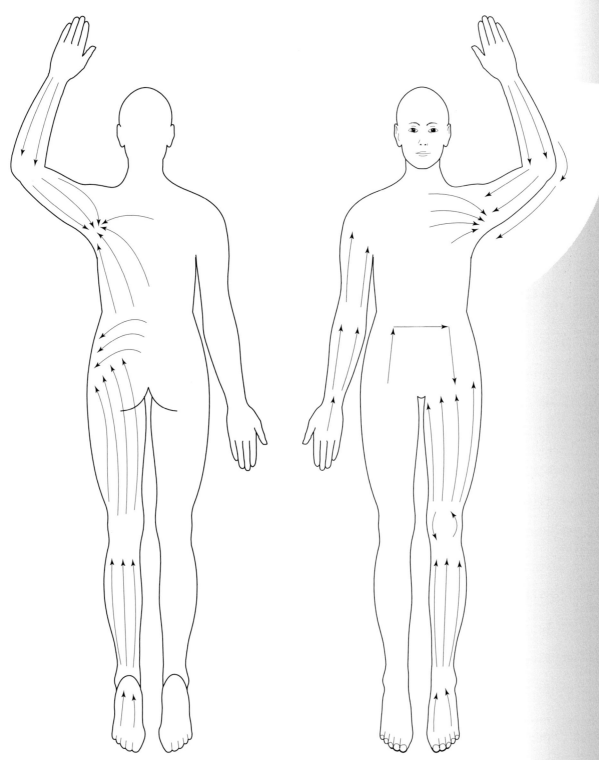

Figure 9.29 Body brushing strokes, prone lying position.

Figure 9.30 Body brushing strokes, supine lying position.

◎ Ask her/him to tell you if s/he feels uncomfortable at any time during the treatment

◎ You may apply talcum powder to the area before treatment but some therapists feel that this is unnecessary

◎ Cover with clean towels the areas not being worked on.

Procedure

◎ Place the client in the prone position with arms above the head (forming a Y shape)

◎ Stand facing the foot

◎ Brush up the sole of the foot from the toes to the heel

◎ Follow each brush stroke with a hand stroke

◎ Brush from ankle to popliteal fossa, in three strips: medial, middle and lateral. Follow with hand strokes

◎ Brush from knee over the buttocks into inguinal nodes, hand strokes

◎ Brush from sacrum up side of spine over shoulder, hand strokes

◎ Brush one brush width away from spine into axilla, hand strokes

◎ Brush one brush width away from last stroke into axilla. Continue until whole back is covered.

Turn your body to face the head.

◎ Brush back of hand to elbow, hand strokes

◎ Brush from elbow into axilla, hand strokes.

Repeat all movements on the other side of the body.

Place client in supine position (face up)

◎ Brush down foot to ankle, hand strokes

◎ Brush from ankle to patella, hand strokes

◎ Brush medial and lateral aspect of knee, hand strokes

◎ Brush from knee into inguinal nodes (use very light strokes on the medial aspect of the thigh), hand strokes

◎ Brush abdomen up ascending colon on right side, across transverse colon under ribs, and down descending colon on left, hand strokes

◎ Brush very lightly from sternum to axilla, hand strokes (avoid breast area)

◎ Brush hand up to elbow, hand strokes

◎ Brush from elbow to axilla, hand strokes.

Contra-indications

➤ any skin diseases or disorders

➤ bruises

➤ infections or open wounds

➤ very thin skin on older clients

➤ varicose veins (prominent)

➤ thrombosis or phlebitis

➤ skin tags and warts

➤ pigmented, raised moles

➤ very thin, bony clients

➤ recent scar tissue

➤ extensive areas of dilated capillaries.

Body polishing

There are many products on the market for body exfoliation and polishing. The palms of the hands are used to spread the product and to apply friction to the skin in circular or short stroking movements. Some manufacturers recommend the use of cleansing products for use before polishing, and oils for massage after polishing. Read the instructions for the use of the product carefully and study the ingredients. These products, like the massage lubricants, can cause allergic reactions: always be alert to any contra-actions.

Treatment technique

◎ Prepare the client as previously explained

◎ With the client in the prone position, stand level with the knee

◎ Spread the product lightly over your palms and apply it to the calf and thigh. With one hand on the calf and the other on the thigh, use small circular movements and short stroking movements to loosen the dead skin cells. Work evenly covering the whole area thoroughly

◎ Repeat on other leg

◎ Remove the product and loosened skin with a warm damp towel. Work neatly, folding back the towel as each area is cleaned

◎ Cover the legs with a clean towel.

Uncover the back.

◎ Apply the product over the back from the sacrum to the shoulders

◎ Work on either side of the spine with circular and short stroking movements to loosen the dead skin cells. Work upwards and outwards over the shoulders; work down the sides and in and out until the back is well covered

◎ Remove the product with a warm damp towel, begin on outside and work inwards. Fold back the towel as each area is cleaned

◎ Cover the back with a clean towel.

Help the client to turn over and cover her/him with towels.

◎ Treat front of legs the same as the back of legs but pay extra attention to the knee area

◎ Uncover the abdomen, apply the product and use circular movements all over. Begin above pubic bone and work out to the sides and down the centre, cover well

◎ Remove the product as for the back

◎ Cover the abdomen with a clean towel

◎ Uncover the sternum and bust. Work gently in this region as the skin may be particularly delicate

◎ Apply the product over the area but avoid the nipple

◎ Work with small circular movements. Begin with the pads of the fingers at the sternum under the clavicle, and work out over the shoulders and back to sternum. Repeat until the area is well covered

◎ Remove the product with warm damp towel and cover with clean towel

◎ Cover the chest

◎ Work on each arm in turn

◎ Support the arm with one hand under the elbow and apply the product and friction with the other hand all over the upper arm

◎ Move down to support at the wrist and repeat over forearm

◎ Remove with warm damp towel and cover

◎ Move to the other side and repeat over other arm

◎ Wash your hands to remove all the product.

The client may then shower or receive massage with appropriate oil, lotion or cream.

QUESTIONS

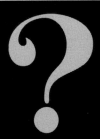

1. Name two changes in muscle tissue that indicate increased tension.
2. List four causes of musculo-skeletal problems.
3. State why massage should not be used in the acute stage of injury.
4. Give two non-verbal responses that will indicate to you that the client is in pain.
5. Briefly explain the physiological changes that occur as a result of prolonged increase in muscle tension.
6. Give two ways in which you would differentiate between fibrous nodules and fatty nodules.
7. Complete the following sentences:
   (a) Superficial pressure is used to palpate......... tissues.
   (b) .... pressure is used to palpate deeper tissues.
8. Give two signs that will indicate the presence of a trigger point.
9. Briefly explain why knowledge of muscle shape and fibre direction is important while performing neuromuscular stroking techniques.
10. List the four techniques that may be used for myofascial release.
11. Define the term 'passive movement'.
12. List any six questions that you would ask the client during consultation, to ensure that there are no joint problems, before performing passive movement.
13. List six contra-indications to passive movement.
14. Explain briefly why thrombosis or phlebitis are contra-indications to passive movement.
15. List six effects of passive movement.
16. State why it is important to know the anatomy and direction of movement of each joint.
17. Complete the following: Each joint should be moved through .... without applying force.
18. Name the movements possible at the elbow joint.
19. Name one other joint that has the same movements as the elbow joint.
20. Give two examples of a ball and socket joint.

10 Mechanical massage

OBJECTIVES

After you have studied this chapter you will be able to:
1. distinguish between the different types of mechanical massage equipment
2. distinguish between the effects produced by the different types of equipment and the various 'heads'
3. select the appropriate massage equipment to suit the needs of the client
4. identify any contra-indications to the treatment
5. treat the client, paying due consideration to maximum efficiency, comfort, safety and hygiene.

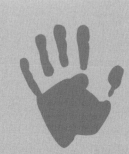

Mechanical massage is the manipulation of body tissues using machines. Generally, mechanical massage is used in conjunction with other treatments to relieve muscle tension and muscle pain, to improve the circulation and to improve certain skin conditions. Provided the client is on a reducing diet, the heavier vibrations may help to disperse fatty deposits from specific areas of the body.

Many different types of appliance are manufactured to produce effects similar to those of a manual massage. They vary from the small hand-held percussion and audio-sonic equipment designed to treat small, localised areas, to the large heavy gyratory vibrators used for deeper effects on large areas of the body. Although the effects are similar to those of manual massage, the sensation felt by the client is very different. The treatment is rather impersonal and the use of a machine rather than the touch of hands is not as pleasing to the client.

In practice, most mechanical vibratory treatments should be combined with some manual massage, thus gaining the more personal aspects of manual massage combined with the depth and power of vibratory equipment. Using mechanical massage equipment is certainly less tiring for the therapist than performing a long, vigorous manual massage. The effects produced are similar for all types of massage equipment, but are deeper and greater with the heavier machines. The treatment is very popular with clients, as they feel invigorated and consider that the desired results will be achieved.

❖ *Gyratory vibrator* ❖

Massage with this type of appliance is much heavier than with percussion and audio-sonic vibrators. It is therefore more suitable for heavier work on large and bulky areas of the body. There are two main types of appliance.

1 **The hand-held vibrator**: this is heavy to use as all the electrical component parts are held in the hand. It is useful for domiciliary work.

2 **The floor-standing vibrator**, commonly called G5: this is a very popular treatment in the salon. Here all the electrical components are housed in a box, which is supported by a stand, and only the moving head is held in the hand. This machine uses a rotary electric motor to turn a crank, which is attached to the head. The head is driven to turn in gyratory motion, moving round and round, up and down and side to side with pressure, providing a deep massage. A variety of attachments is available, which screw onto the head; they are designed to simulate the movements of manual massage:

a) effleurage: sponge heads, curved and disc

b) petrissage: hard rubber heads, single and double ball, flat disc, four half-ball (eggbox), multi-hard spike

c) tapotement: fine spiky and brush heads.

Treatment Technique
Preparation of the client

1 Place the client in a well-supported comfortable position.

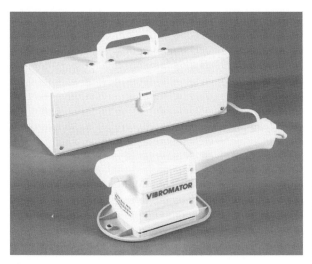
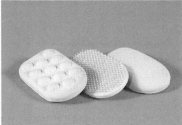

Figure 10.1 Hand-held vibrator and heads.

2 Check that all jewellery has been removed.

3 Check for contra-indications.

4 Clean the skin with cologne.

5 Explain the treatment to the client.

6 Select the appropriate pre-heating treatment.

7 Apply talcum powder to the area using effleurage strokes (do not use oil as it may cause deterioration of the sponge heads).

Procedure

1 Select the appropriate heads to suit the needs of the client. Do not change the heads too often as this breaks the continuity of the treatment.

a) **Effleurage**: use curved sponge on limbs or round sponge elsewhere.

b) **Kneading**: use the flat disc head for lighter petrissage; the four-ball head for deeper petrissage; the multi-hard spike for very deep petrissage on very heavy areas of adipose tissue; and the single and double ball heads on specific, localised areas.

c) **Desquamation**: use fine spiky and brush heads.

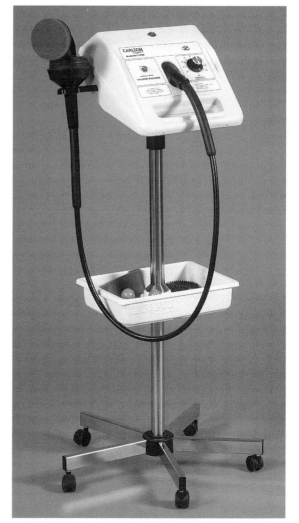

Figure 10.2   Floor-standing gyratory vibrator.

To maintain high standards of hygiene, the heads can be placed in a plastic bag, which should be changed for each client.

2 Switch the machine on, holding the head below the level of the couch. (This is a safety precaution in case the head is insecure – if it flies off it will not hit the client.)

3 With the sponge applicator, apply in long sweeping strokes following the direction of venous return and natural contours of the body. The stroke should be light and smooth rather than abrupt and jerky. The pressure should be heavier on muscle bulk. Cover the area well.

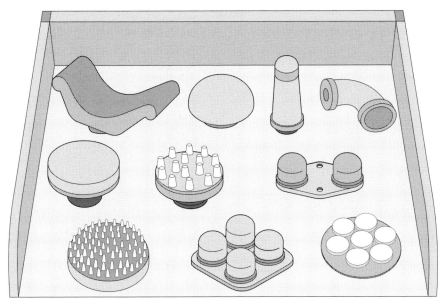

Figure 10.3   Examples of different heads for the gyratory vibrator.

4 Change the head for kneading. Use a circular kneading motion, using the other hand to support the tissues and lift them towards the head. Again apply upward pressure and work with venous return. Cover the area well.

5 Keep the surface of the attachment parallel to the surface of the body at all times. (If one side lifts off the body, there is a danger of damaging the tissues with the hard edge of the head.)

6 Change to the effleurage head to complete the treatment.

7 The degree of erythema and client tolerance dictates the length of the treatment.

8 Wash the heads in hot water and detergent, and allow them to dry.

Note: particular care should be taken when selecting heads for treating the abdominal wall. Abdominal organs have no bony framework for protection – their only protection is provided by the muscles and tissues of the abdominal wall. Overstretched muscles with poor tone offer less protection. This must be considered when treating the abdomen. The heavier petrissage heads should only be used on well-toned abdominal muscles with a covering of adipose tissue, e.g. the younger, overweight client.

Effects

1 As with manual massage, the main effect is stimulation of the circulation. The movements speed up the flow of blood in the veins, removing deoxygenated blood and waste

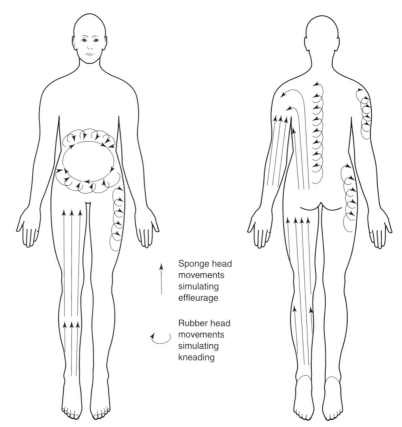

Sponge head
movements
simulating
effleurage

Rubber head
movements
simulating
kneading

Figure 10.4   Direction of strokes for gyratory vibrator.

products more rapidly. This affects the arterial circulation, bringing oxygenated blood and nutrients to the area. Lymph drainage via the lymphatic vessels is also increased.

2 Increased blood supply will increase the metabolic rate in the tissues. This will improve the condition of the tissues.

3 Increased blood supply and friction of the heads will raise the temperature of the area and therefore aid muscle relaxation and relieve pain.

4 Pain in muscles may also be relieved due to rapid removal of waste products, such as lactic acid.

5 Surface capillaries dilate giving an erythema. This improves skin tone.

6 The desquamating effect of the heads may improve the texture of the skin.

7 The continuous heavy pressure on adipose tissue and increased circulation to the area may aid the dispersion of fatty deposits if the client is on a reducing diet.

Uses

The gyratory vibrator is used:

| 1 | for spot reduction of fatty deposits in conjunction with other treatments and reduced food intake |

| 2 | to relieve muscular tension |

| 3 | to reduce muscular aches and pains |

| 4 | to improve poor circulation |

| 5 | to improve the texture of dry, flaky, rough skin. |

Contra-indications

| 1 | skin diseases and disorders |

| 2 | bruises |

| 3 | dilated capillaries |

| 4 | varicose veins |

| 5 | thrombosis or phlebitis |

| 6 | skin tags, warts or pigmented moles |

| 7 | recent operations and scar tissue |

| 8 | treatment of the abdomen during pregnancy and menstruation |

| 9 | extremely hairy areas |

| 10 | thin, bony clients |

| 11 | elderly clients with thin, crêpy skin and lack of subcutaneous fat |

| 12 | acute back and spinal problems, e.g. disc trouble. |

Dangers

Heavy and prolonged treatments can cause bruising and dilated capillaries.

Precautions

1 Check for contra-indications.

2 Do not use heavy percussion over bony areas or over the abdomen with poor muscle tone.

3 Do not over-treat one area: keep the head moving.

4 Keep the head surface parallel to the surface of the body and adapt to body contours.

5 Hold the head away from the client when switching on in case the head is insecure and becomes detached. Hold the head below the bed for safety.

6 Cover the heads with a plastic bag, which can be changed for each client, for hygienic reasons.

❖ *Percussion vibrator* ❖

This is a hand-held appliance: it is lightweight, easy to use and transport. As its name suggests, it is similar in effect to manual percussion movements. An electric motor is used to make the head move or tap up and down on the skin. The head can be fitted with a variety of attachments, e.g. sponge or spike. Some percussion vibrators have an adjustment knob for increasing and decreasing the intensity of the tap. As the knob is tightened, the tap intensity decreases; as the knob is released, the tap intensity increases. This should be carefully controlled to suit the tissues being treated. The number of movements per second is constant, relating to the frequency of the current. With mains frequency of 50 Hz (cycles per second), each tap occurs every half cycle, therefore the rate of tapping will be 100 per second. The treatment time may vary from 5–15 minutes depending on the desired effects. It is used mainly on the face, neck and across the shoulders.

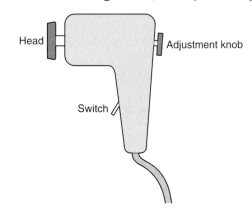

Figure 10.5   Percussion vibrator.

❖ *Audio-sonic vibrator* ❖

This is another type of hand-held appliance. Its name is derived from the fact that the machine produces a humming sound (it should not be confused with ultrasound therapy, which is quite different). This vibrator uses an electromagnet. When the current is passing one way, the coil moves forward; as the current reverses, the coil moves back. This movement forward and backward is transmitted to the head of the appliance. When the head is placed on the tissues, the forward–backward movement of the coil alternately compresses and decompresses the tissues.

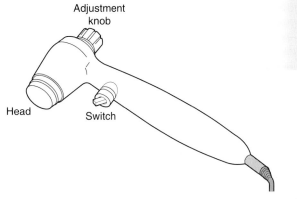

Figure 10.6   Audio-sonic vibrator.

Because the head does not physically move forward and backward, this appliance has a gentler action than the percussion vibrator. It penetrates more deeply into the tissues, but is less stimulating on the surface of the skin. It is, therefore, more suitable for use on sensitive areas of the face and on a mature skin. It is particularly useful for relaxing tension nodules.

Treatment technique for percussion and audio-sonic vibrators

Preparation of the client

1. Place the client in a well-supported and comfortable position.

2. Check that all jewellery has been removed.

3. Check for contra-indications.

4. Explain the treatment to the client.

5. Cleanse the skin.

6. Apply talcum powder for oily/normal skin or cream for dry skin. (Read the manufacturer's instructions.)

Procedure

1. Select the appropriate head and secure it firmly to the vibrator.

2. Switch the machine on away from the client.

3. Commence the treatment using straight lines or a circular motion; ensure coverage of all areas, but avoid delicate areas around the eyes and prominent cheek-bones.

4 The skin reaction indicates the length of the treatment time. When an even erythema is produced, the treatment should stop. This may take from 5 to 15 minutes.

5 The vibrator can be used indirectly over bony or sensitive areas, e.g. cheek-bones and forehead. The therapist places her/his hand between the face and the vibrator head. This reduces the stimulation.

6 Remove the talcum powder or cream and complete the facial routine.

7 Clean the heads, wash with hot water and detergent and disinfect with surgical wipes. Brushes and sponges may be soaked in disinfectant.

Effects

1 It produces an increase in circulation to the treated area, bringing nutrients and oxygen to the area and removing waste products. This improves the condition of the tissues.

2 It produces vasodilation, giving hyperaemia and erythema, improving the colour and tone of the skin.

3 It increases the metabolic rate, thus improving the condition of the tissues.

4 The increase in circulation and the friction of the heads raise the temperature of the area. This promotes relaxation, relieves pain and may stimulate the activity of sebaceous glands.

5 The friction of the heads aids desquamation: this removes the surface layer of cells, improving the condition of the skin.

Uses

Percussion and audio-sonic vibrators are used:

1 to stimulate dry, dehydrated or mature skin: the improved circulation and increase in metabolic rate will improve the condition of the skin

2 to stimulate sebaceous glands: the warmth generated in the tissues will stimulate the production and release of sebum, which will help to lubricate the dry, tired, mature skin

3 to aid desquamation of a sluggish skin: the friction of the heads on the body part will aid the removal of the surface layer, improving texture of the skin

4 to improve and maintain the condition of normal skin

5 to promote relaxation of muscle fibres: the warmth produced in the area will aid relaxation and relieve tension. It is particularly effective over localised tension nodules.

Contra-indications

1 any skin diseases or inflammatory disorders

2 infected acne

3 highly vascular or telangiectatic skin or dilated capillaries

4 sinus problems

5 headaches or migraines

6 lean bony features

7 mature skin with poor elasticity.

Precautions

1 Check for contra-indications.

2 Do not use over very bony areas.

3 Avoid the eye region.

4 Keep the head surface parallel to the surface of the face.

5 Do not over-treat one area – keep the head moving.

❖ *Heat treatment* ❖

There are two types of lamp used for heating the tissues:

1 infra-red lamps, which are non-luminous

2 radiant heat lamps, which are luminous or glowing.

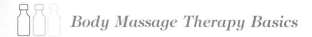

Uses

1 As a general heating treatment to promote relaxation

2 As a localised treatment for relief of pain and tension

3 As a preheating treatment, either generally or locally, to increase the circulation and thus make following treatments more effective.

Effects of infra-red heat
Heating of body tissues

When infra-red rays are absorbed by the tissues, heat is produced in the area. The rays from luminous generators penetrate more deeply than those from non-luminous lamps. Penetration is approximately 3 mm of tissue, therefore superficial and deeper tissues are heated directly.

With non-luminous lamps the top 1 mm of skin is heated directly, but the deeper tissues are heated by conduction.

Increased metabolic rate

(Van't Hoff's law states that a chemical reaction capable of being accelerated will be accelerated by heat.)

Metabolism is a chemical change that will be accelerated by heat. The increase in metabolic rate will be greatest where the heating is greatest, i.e. in the superficial tissues; therefore more oxygen and nutrients are required and more waste products and metabolites are produced.

Vasodilation with increase in circulation

Heat has a direct effect on the blood vessels, producing vasodilation and an increase in blood flow in an attempt to cool the area. Vasodilation is also produced by stimulation of sensory nerve endings, which causes reflex dilation of arterioles.

Fall in blood pressure

If the superficial blood vessels dilate, the peripheral resistance is reduced and this will result in a fall in blood pressure. (When blood flows through vessels with small lumen, it exerts a certain pressure on the walls. If the lumen is increased by the vessels' dilating, the pressure on the walls will be reduced.)

Increase in heart rate

The increased metabolism and circulation mean that the heart must beat faster to meet the demand: therefore the heart rate increases.

General rise in body temperature

When one area of the body is heated for a prolonged time, there is a general rise in body temperature by conduction and convection. The heat will spread through surrounding tissues and will be carried by the blood circulating through the area.

Increased activity of sweat glands

As the body temperature rises, the heat-regulating centres in the brain are affected and the sweat glands are then stimulated to produce more sweat in order to lose body heat. This increases the elimination of waste products.

Effects on muscle tissue

Muscle tissue is affected in two ways:

1 The rise in temperature produces muscle relaxation and relieves tension and pain.

2 The increase in circulation provides the nutrients and oxygen necessary for muscle contraction, and the removal of waste is speeded up.

When muscles are warm, they contract more efficiently than when cold.

Effects on sensory nerves

Mild heat has a soothing effect on sensory nerve endings. However, intense heat has an irritating effect.

Pigmentation

Repeated and intense exposure to infra-red produces a purple or brown mottled appearance on the area. This may be due to destruction of blood cells and release of haemoglobin.

CONTRA-INDICATIONS

1 Areas of defective skin sensation and hypersensitive skin.

2 Heart conditions and blood pressure disorders (high or low).

3 Thrombosis or phlebitis or any areas of deficient circulation.

4 Heavy colds and fevers.

5 Migraines and headaches.

6 Skin disorders and diseases.

7 Diabetes, as skin sensitivity may be impaired.

8 Recent scar tissue (defective sensitivity).

9 Extensive bruising.

10 Recent exposure to UVL (sunburn).

11 Body infra-red would not be given in the last four months of pregnancy or first two days of a heavy period.

12 Any area where linaments or ointments have been applied.

13 Recent soft tissue injury.

DANGERS

1 Burns may be caused if the:
   a) heat is too intense
   b) client is too near the lamp and fails to report overheating
   c) skin sensation is defective and the client may not be aware of overheating
   d) client touches the lamp
   e) lamp should fall and touch the client, or the bedding; overheating of pillows and blankets can cause fire and burns.

2 Electric shock from faulty apparatus or water near the treatment area, producing a short circuit.

3 Headache due to irradiating the back of the neck and head or overheating by prolonged exposure.

4 Faintness due to overheating or extensive irradiation, which may cause a fall in blood pressure, making the client feel faint.

5 Damage to the eyes: infra-red exposure of the eyes can cause cataracts; a client should close her/his eyes and turn away from the lamp, wear goggles or have cotton wool over her/his eyes.

6 Chill may occur if the client goes out into the cold too quickly after exposure.

PRECAUTIONS

1 Clean the skin with cologne to remove sebum.

2 Ensure a safe distance of the lamp from the client. This distance depends on the client's tolerance and the output of the lamp (45–90 cm).

3 Do not place the lamp directly over the client.

4 Ensure that the lamp is stable with the head over a foot if lamp has three or five feet.

5 Ensure that the lamp is in good working order and that there are no dents in the reflector.

6 Ensure that the flexes are sound and not trailing in a walking area.

7 Check for contra-indications.

8 Carry out a hot and cold sensitivity test (see as follows).

9 Protect the eyes.

10 Explain the importance of calling immediately if the client feels too hot, faint, nauseous or uncomfortable.

11 Warn the client not to move nearer to or touch the lamp.

12 The client should rest after treatment and not get up too quickly.

Treatment technique
Preparation of the client

1 Place the client in a comfortable position (when treating areas of the back, use side lying or the recovery position, well supported by pillows. If treating knees use half lying).

2 Check that all jewellery has been removed.

3 Clean the area with cologne to remove sebum.

4 Check for contra-indications.

5 Explain the treatment to the client.

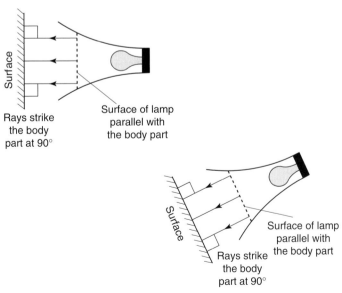

Figure 10.7   Positioning of the lamp.

6   Carry out a sensitivity test using two test tubes, one filled with hot water and the other filled with cold water. Instruct the client to close her/his eyes. Carry out the test all over the area to be irradiated. Touch the client with either the hot test tube or the cold test tube at random over the area. Ask her/him if s/he feels hot or cold. (If the client cannot tell the difference between the hot and the cold, s/he has defective sensation, and the treatment should not be carried out.)

7   Cover the areas not receiving treatment.

8   Warn the client that warmth should be comfortable and to call if the heat becomes too intense.

9   Warn the client not to touch the lamp or move too close to it.

PROCEDURE

1   Check the plug, leads and reflector.

2   Switch the lamp on directed at the floor.
   a) IR takes 10–15 minutes to reach maximum output.
   b) Radiant heat (visible) takes around 2 minutes.

3   When maximum intensity is reached, position the lamp ensuring stability. (If the lamp has three feet, place the head of the lamp over one of the feet, ensuring that the angle joints are secure.)

4   Make sure that the face of the lamp is parallel with the part so that the rays strike the part at 90° for maximum penetration, absorption and effect. Do not place the lamp directly above the client. (This also applies if infra-red rays are being used as a preheating treatment.)

5   Select an appropriate distance between 45–90 cm. The selected distance depends on two factors:
   a) the intensity of the lamp
   b) the client's tolerance (60 cm) is a good average.

6   Ensure that the rays are not irradiating the client's face. (The lamp should not be irradiating the eyes or the face of the client nor the therapist.) If using infra-red rays for facial work, the client's eyes must be closed and covered with cotton wool.

7   Observe the client throughout the treatment.

8   Treatment time is 15–20 minutes, until the desired effect is obtained.

9   The treatment may be followed by massage.

(Do not use infra-red before going on a sunbed as the reaction to UVL will be intensified. Infra-red may be used after over-exposure to UVL to reduce the reaction. The client should not rise suddenly after infra-red treatment, as the blood pressure is lowered and the client may feel faint.)

POINTS TO CONSIDER WHEN POSITIONING THE LAMP

1 Ensure a safe but effective distance from the part.

2 Never place the lamp directly over the client. If it falls or the bulb breaks, it would cause burns to the client.

3 Position the lamp so that the surface of the lamp is parallel to the part and the rays strike the part at 90° for maximum penetration, absorption and effect. This applies whenever the lamp is used.

4 Avoid the face and eyes.

Q U E S T I O N S

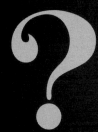

1. Give three uses for mechanical massage on the body.
2. Name three different types of mechanical massage equipment.
3. List four contra-indications to mechanical massage on the body.
4. List the effects of mechanical massage on the body.
5. Explain briefly why audio-sonic vibrators have an advantage over percussion vibrators on a sensitive area.
6. Give four effects of percussion vibrator treatment to the face.
7. Give two different uses for each of the following:
   (a) gyratory vibrator (G5)
   (b) percussion vibrator
   (c) audio-sonic vibrator.
8. Explain briefly how you would incorporate mechanical massage into a body treatment routine.
9. Give reasons why the heavy gyratory vibrator heads should not be used on the abdominal wall of certain clients.
10. Explain the procedure for maintaining high standards of hygiene when using gyratory vibrators.
11. Explain briefly why a sensitivity test must be carried out before an infra-red treatment.
12. Give the two factors that govern the choice of distance when giving infra-red treatment.
13. Explain why blood pressure will fall when the client has infra-red treatment.
14. Give four dangers of infra-red treatment.

11 Introduction to sports massage

OBJECTIVES

After you have studied this chapter you will be able to:
1. explain the benefits of sports massage
2. list the four categories where massage is used in sport
3. explain the objectives of each category
4. perform the suggested techniques for each category
5. explain the effects of the massage routines in each category.

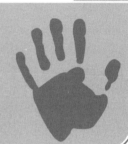

The field of sport or athletic massage is highly specialised and should not be undertaken by anyone without appropriate training. A qualification in massage is not enough. Additional knowledge and practice under the supervision of an experienced sports massage therapist is required. Further study of anatomy and physiology, with particular emphasis on those systems affected by exercise, is needed. A study of kinesiology (body movement), biomechanics (scientific principles relating to movement) and an understanding of the requirements of the different sports or athletic activities are also necessary.

This in-depth knowledge and understanding will enable the massage therapist to carry out an assessment and provide appropriate treatment for the wide variety of conditions that s/he will encounter. To be effective, the therapist must have empathy and rapport with the performer and the coach or trainer. S/he must be part of the training team, giving advice and explaining the effects and benefits of massage as appropriate. The therapist's knowledge and professionalism must inspire confidence.

❖ *Training* ❖

Athletes or sportspeople are highly trained, finely tuned individuals who are usually totally focused on achieving success in their particular field. They will train and stress the body to its limit, i.e. to the point of breakdown. They may train too hard and too frequently in an effort to improve performance. Hard training with inadequate rest periods to allow full recovery will result in a decline in performance and leave the body vulnerable to serious injury.

As a result of over-training and incomplete recovery, the athlete may suffer from any of the following symptoms: vague aches and pains; acute pain in muscles, bones or joints; inflammation of tendons, ligaments or bursae resulting in pain and swellings; and symptoms of stress such as headaches, listlessness, tension, insomnia or increased irritability.

Athletes and their trainers should be made aware that hard training must be balanced with rest periods to allow adequate or full recovery of the tissues and to restore homeostasis (body balance). The harder and longer the training, the longer the rest period should be. If homeostasis is not restored and tissue recovery is incomplete, then the level of performance will eventually decline. Massage following training and performance will greatly hasten the recovery of the tissues. Research indicates that recovery is four to five times faster in tissues receiving massage than in those simply allowed to rest. A shorter recovery time allows for a greater number of training sessions, which will improve performance.

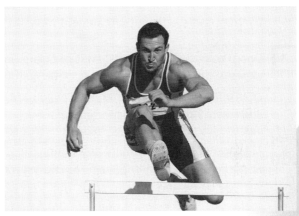

Figure 11.1   A highly trained athlete.

Injuries of the musculo-skeletal system occur as a result of poor technique and over-training. When tired and over-stressed, these structures are more vulnerable to injury. Minor injuries may result in greater injury or serious damage if ignored or neglected. The massage therapist will detect areas of tension and abnormalities within the tissues. Appropriate treatment and rest in these initial stages will prevent further damage.

When injuries occur, they must be referred to a medical practitioner for accurate diagnosis and appropriate treatment. The rate of recovery and return to full function will depend on these factors. Inappropriate treatment or inadequate recovery time may result in further damage and permanently impaired function.

❖ *Benefits of sports massage* ❖

1 Massage increases the blood flow through the area being massaged, i.e. it produces hyperaemia. The delivery of nutrients and oxygen is therefore increased. These are required for muscle contraction and also to aid recovery of the muscles and maintain them in good condition.

2 Massage generates heat in the tissues through the friction of the hands moving over the surface; through the friction between the tissues as they move over one another; through the dilation of vessels and capillaries, which allows more warm blood to flow through the part. Warmth increases the metabolic rate, which will improve the condition of the tissues. Warmth also improves flexibility of the tissues, muscle fibres, fascia, tendons and ligaments, which are therefore less prone to strains and sprains. Warm muscles contract more efficiently than cold muscles.

3 Deep massage movements exert pressure on the tissues, which increases the permeability of cell membranes. This facilitates the exchange of tissue fluids between cells and vessels. Nutrients and oxygen are transported into the cells more efficiently and waste products transported out.

4 Massage speeds up venous and lymphatic drainage from the area, which removes the waste products of metabolism. Following training or performance, the waste products such as lactic and pyruvic acids build up within the muscle, producing pain and stiffness. The increased pressure produced by these acids also interferes with the recovery of the muscle. Massage flushes these substances out of the muscles, thus reducing pain and stiffness and speeding up muscle recovery. Speedy recovery allows the athlete to fit in more training, which will raise the standard of performance.

5 Massage increases the flexibility of the tissues. Stretching manipulations such as wringing and muscle rolling move the tissues transversely. This stretches the muscle fibres and fascial compartments to a greater extent than the longitudinal pull of stretch exercises. Muscles are also lifted and moved over supporting structures, muscle bundles are separated and fascial compartments are stretched. This greatly increases flexibility and extensibility, which will improve performance and reduce the risk of injury.

6 Massage provides an early warning system to the risk of potential injury. Areas of tightness or tension may be detected in the course of a massage. Appropriate stretch manipulations and exercise can then be advised to overcome the problem and restore flexibility.

7 Massage will break down or stretch inflexible scar tissue found in muscles, tendons or ligaments of the sportsperson. These may be the result of past injuries or over-use. Scar tissue is part of the healing process and is laid down between the torn parts. It forms a tight inflexible mass that interferes with the normal function of the muscles or ligaments. Deep, short stroking movements or frictions will break down, or improve the flexibility of, this tissue, thus restoring function.

8 Massage will break down adhesions within the muscles. Exudate is part of the inflammatory healing process. If it is not quickly absorbed it becomes sticky and binds down the tissues, causing them to stick to one another. Deep friction will loosen and free these structures, allowing muscles and tendons to function normally.

9 Massage around joints will improve the circulation and generate warmth. This will improve the condition of joints and maintain the flexibility of joint structures. Frictions around the joint will break down adhesions from old traumas and free ligaments to function normally.

10 Massage improves flexibility and elasticity of hard, bulky, inelastic muscles following hard isometric exercise training. These exercises impede the free flow of blood to the muscle, which slows down the metabolic rate. The condition of the muscle deteriorates, which reduces the level of performance. Regular massage and other forms of training will prevent this deterioration.

11 Massage will promote local or general relaxation. The warmth generated in the tissues will aid relaxation. The fast removal of metabolic waste will prevent pain and stiffness developing, thus relieving tension. The rhythmic stretching manipulations promote relaxation. Slow rhythmical massage has a soothing effect on the nervous system. These movements produce a reflex response, which releases tension. General massage also has an effect on the autonomic nervous system, which improves relaxation.

❖ *Use of massage in sport* ❖

Massage may be used in four distinct categories to help sportspeople. Although all the basic massage manipulations may be used, certain considerations and adaptations must be made. It is important that athletes and their trainers are aware of these differences and appreciate their effects.

Massage may be given in the following instances:

- ➤ before an event or performance (pre-event massage)
- ➤ after an event or performance (post-event massage)
- ➤ as part of the training programme (training massage)
- ➤ as a rehabilitation treatment (treatment massage).

❖ *Pre-event massage* ❖

The aim of this massage is to help the body respond to the demands of increased activity and facilitate optimum performance. The objectives are to:

- ◎ increase the delivery of nutrients and oxygen to the contracting muscles
- ◎ warm the muscles, thus improving contractility

◎ improve the flexibility and extensibility of muscles

◎ maintain maximum range of movement of joints.

At rest the body is in a balanced state known as homeostasis and the systems of the body must just meet the basic metabolic needs. Muscular activity requires an abundant supply of energy and the body systems must respond rapidly to meet these needs. An increased supply of nutrients and oxygen must be delivered to the working muscles. Warm-up and stretch exercises are essential prior to performance, as they gradually bring the body systems up to a level that will enable the athlete to perform at maximum potential. Massage must not replace these exercises but may be used to enhance their effect.

Treatment technique

This massage must be brisk and of fairly short duration, e.g. 7–10 minutes for each area. It must be stimulating to create alertness and focus. It should concentrate on the body parts involved in the performance, but both sides of the body must be treated to maintain balance. It is usual to include the back with both upper and lower parts of the body. For example, for throwers cover the back, shoulders and arms; for runners cover the back, buttocks and legs.

A relaxing or general body massage should not be given before a performance because the athlete must remain alert and ready for action. The athlete must have experienced massage during training; s/he should not receive the first massage before performance, as timing and rhythm may be affected.

Experienced therapists will develop their own massage routines and make adaptations according to the needs of the athlete. However, for the treatment to be effective, a basic routine is essential. Pre-event massage is similar to the stimulating massage described in Chapter 8. A suggested routine is as follows:

1	work towards the heart, i.e. distal to proximal with pressure upwards
2	brisk effleurage of moderate depth, progressing to greater depth
3	kneading to main muscle groups and around joints
4	wringing to main muscle groups
5	picking up to main muscle groups
6	effleurage
7	light hacking and cupping to large muscles
8	muscle rolling
9	gentle muscle shaking and compression where possible.

Finish the massage with stroking away from the heart, i.e. proximal to distal. This dilates capillaries and encourages the flow of fresh oxygenated blood into the muscles. Many therapists include passive movements of appropriate joints in the routine. This requires great care, very specific knowledge of joint movement and of the athlete's particular sport, and is not within the scope of this book.

Effects

1 Massage speeds up venous drainage and produces dilation of blood vessels and capillaries. This results in more blood flow – hyperaemia, which increases the availability of nutrients and oxygen required for muscle contraction.

2 Squeezing and pressure of the tissues facilitates the exchange of tissue fluids across cell membranes, increasing absorption.

3 Massage creates warmth in the tissues. Warm muscles contract more efficiently and powerfully than cold muscles, which results in better performance.

4 Warm muscles are also more flexible and extensible and are consequently less likely to tear.

5 The petrissage manipulations, such as wringing and picking up, improve the flexibility of muscle fibres and supporting fascia. This also reduces the risk of injury.

6 Massage performed around the joints warms the surrounding structures, thus increasing flexibility. This facilitates the maximum range of movement and reduces the risk of injury.

❖ *Post-event massage* ❖

The aim of this treatment is to promote speedy and complete muscle recovery and to re-establish homeostasis. The objectives are to:

◎ speed up venous and lymphatic drainage of the area and thus remove metabolic waste

◎ increase the delivery of nutrients and oxygen to combat fatigue and aid muscle recovery

◎ prevent or relieve pain and stiffness

◎ relieve tension and promote relaxation

◎ prevent tightening of fascial components and maintain flexibility

◎ identify areas of tenderness or soreness, which may indicate injury

◎ prevent the formation of adhesions and fibrosis.

The energy for prolonged or vigorous muscle contraction is provided initially from stored adenosine triphosphate (ATP) and phosphocreatine, and then by the breakdown of glucose into pyruvic acid by a process known as glycolysis. If the body can maintain an adequate supply of oxygen (as in steady state aerobic exercises), then the pyruvic acid is completely metabolised to carbon dioxide and water. However, if the exercises are aerobic, i.e. vigorous and there is insufficient oxygen, then the pyruvic acid is converted to lactic acid, which gradually builds up within the muscle. This build up of lactic acid increases the pressure within the muscle, producing pain and stiffness. It also compresses vessels and capillaries, restricting the flow of blood, which reduces the availability of nutrients and oxygen, resulting in muscle fatigue and inhibiting the process of recovery.

Treatment technique

This massage should be given as soon as possible after the event and certainly within the first one to two hours. The massage will then be more effective, as the waste build up is removed more quickly and the recovery will be faster. Great care must be taken when giving post-event massage as the muscles may be tender, sore and painful. This is partly due to the pressure of accumulated waste and also due to any injuries or micro-traumas that may have occurred during performance. Very light pressure should be applied initially, becoming deeper as muscle relaxation is felt. As the prime aim is to clear away metabolites, the strokes should begin proximally near the lymph nodes. This congested area is cleared first and the manipulations work downwards, gradually pushing fluids into the cleared areas (this is explained in lymphatic drainage in Chapter 3).

The movements begin with light stroking and effleurage, gentle muscle lifting, rolling and shaking. Kneading, wringing and picking up should not be used until the muscle has relaxed. The flesh will not be soft enough to yield to the pressure, and rubbing the hard muscle will cause pain and increase tension. Changing the pressure over different areas is essential in post-event massage – it must be very light over painful, tense areas, becoming gradually deeper as the muscle is felt to relax. The therapist must develop the ability to sense the condition of the tissues through the hands and adapt the massage accordingly.

1. Begin proximally to clear the upper congested area first.

2. Gentle stroking over the part will give an indication of the condition of the tissues. This will provide feedback on areas of tension, painful spots, tightness and rigidity. Use very light movements initially.

3. Effleurage: begin proximally and work down, one hand width at a time. For example, on the leg begin on the thigh towards the inguinal nodes in

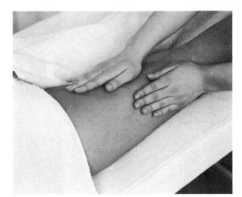

Figure 11.2   Stroking to sense condition of tissues.

the groin – push up, move down one hand width, push up, and so on until the knee is reached. Increase the depth as the muscle relaxes. Keep the movement slow and rhythmic. Then move below the knee and cover the lower leg.

4   Muscle shaking or vibrations: place the flat of the hand on the muscle and gently shake it up and down and from side to side.

5   Muscle rolling: gently grasp and lift the muscle; roll it first to one side and then to the other.

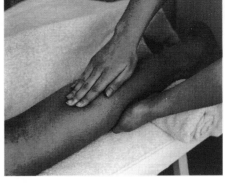

Figure 11.3   Muscle vibrations.

6   Work in this way until the muscles soften and then add any of the following:
   → kneading
   → wringing
   → picking up.

7   Deep stroking: use the tips of the flattened fingers, the heel or the ulnar border of the hand to apply short, deep strokes to the muscle belly to separate the muscle compartments and loosen the fascia.

8   Effleurage from distal to proximal to complete the massage.

Effects

1   Massage speeds up venous and lymphatic drainage of the area. The waste product, lactic acid, is quickly removed, preventing build up within the muscle and thus reducing soreness, pain and stiffness.

2   Massage reduces the pressure and compression created by a build up of metabolic waste and produces dilation of vessels and capillaries. This increases blood flow and the delivery of nutrients and oxygen to the area, reducing muscle fatigue and aiding the recovery of the muscle. Research indicates that recovery is three to four times faster in muscles subjected to massage than in those simply allowed to rest.

3   Gentle massage warms the area and soothes sensory receptors in the skin, reducing tension and inducing relaxation.

4   Stretching manipulations such as muscle rolling, shaking and gentle wringing will maintain the flexibility of the fascia, the extensibility of muscle fibres and the movement of muscle bundles. These stretching effects are important in maintaining overall flexibility.

5 During massage experienced therapists will obtain direct feedback on the condition of the tissues. Through the hands they can sense and become aware of changes within the tissues. Pain, soreness or increased tension are highlighted. These factors may indicate minor traumas that can be immediately treated and allowed to recover, thus preventing more serious injury.

❖ *Training massage* ❖

The aim of this massage is to help the athlete achieve and maintain peak condition, thus maximising performance. This massage is very similar to post-event massage, as its main aim is to clear out the waste products and promote speedy recovery. There are, however, differences that should be noted. The objectives are to:

◎ maintain an efficient circulation and delivery of nutrients and oxygen for nourishing the tissues

◎ quickly remove metabolic waste after a training session

◎ promote fast recovery of the muscles, thus allowing greater frequency of training

◎ prevent any minor injuries becoming more serious and chronic

◎ prevent the formation of scar tissue and to stretch old scar tissue

◎ prevent the formation of adhesions and fibrosis

◎ maintain flexibility or elasticity of muscles, fascia, tendons and ligaments

◎ maintain and improve the range of movement at joints

◎ relieve stress and promote relaxation.

Training massage is probably the most beneficial for the athlete. It should be given, like post-event massage, immediately following activity. This will achieve similar effects in flushing out waste products, aiding the recovery of the muscles and restoring homeostasis. Massage identifies and reduces areas of tension that could lead to serious injury. During hard training massage may be given after every session. If given every day or so, it should be fairly light. The massage should concentrate on the strained used areas, although it is important to treat both sides of the body to maintain balance. It is also important to treat antagonistic muscles equally, as increased tension in the antagonistic muscles will limit performance or leave the muscle vulnerable to injury.

Again an upper body massage including the back, or lower body massage including the back, may be given. In addition a full deep body massage should be given once a week. This reduces stress levels and promotes relaxation. This should be followed by one or two days of rest to allow recovery. A full body massage should not be given immediately before an event. At least four or five days should elapse to allow the athlete fully to recover alertness and focus.

If minor injuries occur during training, they may only become apparent during massage. If left untreated they would leave the body vulnerable to further injury. The therapist is able to identify these areas of pain or tension and treat them immediately, thus preventing more extensive or serious trauma. Many minor injuries may occur during training. The more common and easily treatable are described as follows:

◎ Small tears or micro-traumas may occur within muscles. These will heal with the formation of fibrous scar tissue. The extent of fibrous tissue laid down will depend on the extent of the trauma and the speed of recovery. Scar tissue forms a hard inflexible mass within the muscle, which contracts over time. This reduces the extensibility and flexibility of the muscle, impairing its function. Regular massage will speed up the recovery and reduce the amount of scar tissue laid down. Massage will also maintain the suppleness of old scar tissue already present and prevent it contracting.

◎ The fascia surrounding and lying between muscles may tighten as a result of injuries or repetitive strain. This will produce pain and stiffness, which will inhibit muscle action. Stretching massage will separate these fascial compartments, loosen the fascia and release the muscles to function correctly.

◎ Massage around joints will improve nourishment and maintain flexibility of joint structures. The tendons or ligaments around joints may be damaged or over-stretched (sprains) during training or performance. During the healing process, the exudate that is part of the inflammatory process may become tacky and sticky, and form adhesions that bind the tendons and ligaments to underlying structures. Frictions performed around the joint or across the tendons will help to free these structures and restore joint function.

◎ Some forms of training, such as strength training, result in bulky inflexible muscles. Massage will be very beneficial in maintaining the suppleness of these muscles. Use of isometric work, where the muscles contract but do not change in length, inhibits the flow of blood as there is no pumping action on the blood vessels. If there are insufficient rest periods, pressure is maintained on the capillary beds, further restricting blood flow, and muscle fatigue develops quickly. Massage is therefore particularly beneficial following hard isometric training.

Athletes who receive massage during the training sessions recover more quickly and can train more frequently. Many athletes suffer a high degree of stress and anxiety. A general body massage performed regularly once a week can improve the well-being of the athlete. The stress and anxiety levels are reduced, which will relieve symptoms such as headaches, irritability, listlessness and vague aches and pains, and can restore good sleep patterns.

Treatment technique
Training massage should be given regularly as part of the training schedule. It may be a full body massage or it may concentrate on the upper or lower half of the body, depending on the areas of greater stress. A half body massage will take approximately half an hour. A full body

massage of up to one hour may be given once a week, provided it is not within five days or so of an event. For a half body massage begin on the side that has received more stress, but be sure to treat the other side as well. The massage can vary according to the preference of the therapist and the needs of the athlete. The following is one example of a suitable routine:

Upper body

Supine	Prone
◎ arm	◎ arm
◎ shoulder	◎ back
◎ chest	◎ upper
◎ arm	back and
	shoulder
	◎ arm

Lower body

Supine	Prone
◎ thigh	◎ thigh
◎ lower leg	◎ calf
◎ foot	◎ foot
◎ lower leg	◎ calf
◎ thigh	◎ thigh
	◎ buttocks
	◎ back

Use the following manipulations:

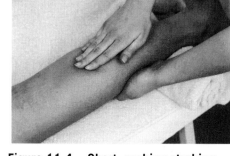

Figure 11.4   Short, probing stroking.

1 superficial stroking: this must be a light, sensitive exploratory movement from distal to proximal in order to introduce the massage and sense the condition of the tissues

2 effleurage: this must be light to moderate if the muscles are sore and tense, becoming deeper if the muscles relax; begin proximally

3 shaking: along the muscle to aid relaxation

4 kneading: if the muscle is soft enough

5 short stroking: to explore and release tense areas. Begin proximally (e.g. just below the groin on the thigh), use the pads of the fingers to probe upwards deeply into the tissues, move down to the next area and repeat. Cover the thigh down to the knee in this way. Where areas of tightness and tension are felt, probe transversally back and forth

6 muscle rolling: lift the muscle and push from side to side from thumbs to fingers and back

7 wringing

8 double-handed pressure kneading (or thumb kneading on anterior tibials). If tightness or nodules are felt in the muscle, ease the pressure

9 shaking

10 effleurage: work down to the foot and then back up with deeper pressure.

Effects

1 Massage improves the circulation to the areas being worked on. The delivery of nutrients and oxygen is increased, thus improving the condition of the muscle and facilitating recovery.

2 Venous and lymphatic drainage are speeded up and metabolic waste is quickly removed from the tissues. This reduces pain and stiffness, which would result from a build up of lactic acid. Recovery time is shorter and therefore more frequent training sessions may be undertaken.

3 The therapist gains feedback on the condition of the tissues during massage. Minor injuries may be quickly identified and treated, preventing more serious injuries occurring.

4 Massage reduces the formation of scar tissue following muscle tears. It also immobilises and stretches old scar tissue, improving flexibility of the muscle.

5 Massage removes the sticky exudate following injury. This in turn reduces the formation of adhesions and frees affected structures so that they function correctly.

6 Massage maintains the flexibility of fascia and fascial compartments, enabling the muscles to function efficiently.

7 Frictions around the joints will loosen and release bound ligaments, improving joint range.

8 Massage relieves pressure and rigidity within muscle groups following isometric exercise and restores muscle elasticity.

❖ *Treatment massage* ❖

The aim of this type of massage is to promote rapid healing and aid complete recovery of the tissues, thus restoring normal function. The objectives are to:

◎ reduce the inflammatory response

◎ promote healing and reduce pain, swelling and stiffness

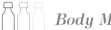

◎ gradually mobilise and stretch the affected tissues

◎ return the body to normal function.

Accurate diagnosis is crucial following injury and the athlete must be seen by a doctor as soon as possible. Those without medical training should not attempt to diagnose or treat sports injuries. However, knowing what action to take immediately before medical attention is available can reduce the extent of tissue damage. Treatment can be given by an experienced therapist if the diagnosis reveals that the injury is of a minor nature, or under the guidance of a medical practitioner.

Treatment technique

Immediate action involves:

R   for rest and immobilisation to prevent further damage
I   for ice, applied immediately for vasoconstriction
C   for compression to the area to reduce swelling
E   for elevation, using gravity to assist drainage of exudate from the area
D   for diagnosis by a doctor, on site, in a surgery or in a hospital.

Rest

Rest is essential for all sudden, acute injuries because continued movement can increase the extent of the damage. Movement may increase bleeding into the tissues; it may increase the inflammatory response with increased fluid exudate and swelling of the tissues; or it may cause further tearing and damage of the muscle fibres, tendons or ligaments. Resting the part may be sufficient, but it is usually necessary to use some form of support such as splints, tubular or stocking supports, crêpe bandages, slings and collars. Care must be taken that the strapping is firm but not too tight, as this can restrict the circulation and cause further damage. The strapping must be able to stretch or give if the swelling increases.

Ice

Ice should be placed over the injured part as soon as possible. Cold will cause constriction of the blood vessels, which will reduce internal bleeding and fluid exudate. This will prevent excessive bleeding and swelling. Cold also reduces the sensitivity of pain receptors and the conductivity of nerves. It numbs the area, reducing muscle spasm and tension.

Care must be taken when applying the ice as there is a risk of producing ice burns if the ice is in direct contact with the skin for some time. A wet towel should be placed on the skin to protect it and the ice placed on top. There are various ways of applying ice – freezer gel packs are the most convenient, but packs of frozen food can also be used. These are placed over the towel and held in place by another towel wrapped around the part, which will also apply compression. Ice cubes can be crushed and placed inside a towel and placed over the area. Injuries to the ankle or wrist can be treated by immersing the injured part in a bucket of iced water. The part should be held in the water for as long as is tolerable, removed for a few minutes and then re-immersed. Ice packs are kept in place for 10–15 minutes and applied every three or four hours initially, decreasing to three times a day as healing progresses.

Cold sprays are commonly used in sport as they are easy to carry and convenient to use. However, they are not as effective as ice packs as they do not cool the deeper tissues. They are effective only on superficial tissues and are not recommended for use on acute traumas. Over-use in an attempt to reach deeper tissues can result in ice burns to the skin.

Compression

Pressure applied to the area will stop the bleeding and reduce the swelling. Crêpe, tubular or stocking bandages may be used to apply pressure. A pad of cotton wool over the area, before applying the bandage, will increase the pressure over the injury. The bandage must extend above and below the injured area and may include the entire limb. The bandaging must not be too tight, as previously explained.

Elevation

The injured part should be supported in elevation wherever possible. Gravity will then assist the drainage of any fluid exudate away from the part. This will reduce stagnation and the formation of sticky exudate, which can bind structures to each other and hamper movement.

Diagnosis

Accurate diagnosis must be obtained as soon as possible, followed by appropriate rehabilitation. This is crucial to full and complete recovery.

Massage in rehabilitation

Massage must not be given immediately after injury as there is a risk of internal bleeding into the tissues. The treatment in the initial stages of acute injury is ice, compression and rest. Ice should be used for the first six to eight days until there is no risk of bleeding and healing is progressing. If the injuries are minor then massage may begin after two to three days. After the ice is removed the area is very gently and lightly stroked in the direction of venous return (towards the heart). If there is swelling present, the part should be elevated so that gravity can assist the drainage.

If the injuries are more serious then ice treatment is continued, but massage is not used for six to eight days until all danger of further bleeding is over and tissue healing is well under way. After six to eight days the same superficial stroking movement is used to 'sense' the condition of the tissues. As the tissues are felt to relax, deeper movements can be applied. Massage must not produce any pain or increased tension within the tissues – the pressure must be reduced or the massage stopped if this occurs. Vibrations and shaking may be used, particularly above and below the injured part.

After eight to ten days some form of heat may be used, i.e. infra-red or heat packs. This can be followed by deeper massage movements such as effleurage, kneading and muscle rolling. Heat must not be used in the initial stages of treatment, as it dilates blood vessels and increases blood flow to the area. When there is no risk of bleeding and when the healing is under way, it is used to promote and hasten the healing process. Gentle heat for 10–15 minutes should be used initially, increasing to around 25 minutes. Do not overheat as this is counter-productive. Heat increases metabolic rate and promotes healing, but overheating is irritating, interferes with metabolism and slows the process of healing.

As the condition of the tissues improves, then deeper massage movements can be added to the previous regime, e.g. deep effleurage, kneading, wringing (to stretch muscle fibres and fascia), muscle rolling (to maintain flexibility), short deep probing stroking (to stretch fibrous tissue), frictions into tight areas (to stretch any adhesions), deep effleurage and light stroking. These movements must only be used if there is no pain. Return to gentle stroking if any pain or tension is evoked by other movements.

Athletes must allow time for full recovery following trauma and must build up the training routine very gradually. If they return too soon or train too hard, serious chronic conditions, which will permanently affect performance, may result.

❖ Contra-indications to sports massage ❖

- ◎ infections or contagious skin diseases
- ◎ open wounds or abrasions
- ◎ internal bleeding or haemorrhage, or any potential risk of bleeding
- ◎ broken bones
- ◎ severe or extensive bruising
- ◎ muscle ruptures
- ◎ tendon or ligament ruptures
- ◎ burns
- ◎ thrombosis or phlebitis
- ◎ bursitis
- ◎ arthritis
- ◎ undiagnosed areas of deep pain
- ◎ tumours.

Q U E S T I O N S

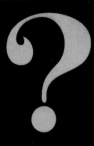

1. Explain six benefits of massage to a sportsperson.
2. Give the four categories where massage would be used.
3. Explain briefly why hard training must be balanced with adequate rest.
4. List any six symptoms that may result from over-training and incomplete rest.
5. Explain what is meant by the term 'homeostasis'.
6. List the objectives of:
   (a) pre-event massage
   (b) post-event massage.
7. Explain the effects of pre-event massage.
8. Explain briefly why lactic acid builds up within a muscle during exercise and how massage helps its removal.
9. Suggest the manipulations you would use for a post-event massage. Give reasons for your selection.
10. Explain why training massage helps the athlete to train more frequently.
11. List six common minor injuries that may occur during training or performance.
12. Give the immediate first aid procedure following injury.
13. Explain why massage should not be given immediately following injury.

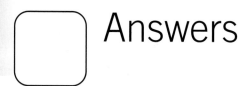

Answers

Answers to questions from Chapter 1: Health, safety and hygiene.

1 a) A hazard is anything that can cause harm.
   b) A risk is the chance, great or small, that someone will be harmed by the hazard.

2 The HSE is a body of people appointed to enforce health and safety law. Their inspectors may inspect your premises at any time.

3 There are four actions that the inspector can take if a breach in the law is found.
   a) Informal notice: for minor problems, the inspector will explain what needs to be done to comply with the regulations.
   b) Improvement notice: if the problem is more serious, corrective action must be taken within a specified time. (At least 21 days must be given for corrective action to be taken.)
   c) Prohibition notice: if the problem poses a serious risk, the inspector will stop the activity immediately and not allow it to resume until corrective action is taken.
   d) Prosecution – if corrective action is not taken in the allocated time the matter may be referred to the courts, who have the power to fine or in severe cases serve imprisonment on those responsible.

4 Take the appropriate corrective action to deal with the hazard and reduce or eliminate the risk. If unable to do so, seek advice from a supervisor or someone able to deal with the situation. Record the hazards identified and the actions taken to rectify them. Inform all colleagues and place the record in a safe place.

5 Any of:
   ➤ adequate ventilation
   ➤ comfortable temperature
   ➤ adequate lighting
   ➤ cleanliness
   ➤ hygiene
   ➤ waste disposal
   ➤ adequate space.

6 Any of the following:
   ➤ maintenance of equipment
   ➤ floors and traffic routes

- ➤ falling objects
- ➤ falls
- ➤ windows.

7 Any of the following:
- ➤ sanitary conveniences
- ➤ drinking water
- ➤ changing rooms
- ➤ facilities for resting.

8 Control of Substances Hazardous to Health.

9 Any of the following: cleaning agents, disinfectants, massage products, powder or dust, micro-organisms, ozone.

10 Suitable and safe for intended use. Inspected regularly by a competent person and maintained in a safe condition. Used only by therapists who are fully informed, trained and competent in their use.

11 Any hazard present in your place of work. For example, a trailing electrical cable is a hazard because there is a risk that staff, clients or other personnel may trip and fall, resulting in injuries.

12 Any of page 23 (Precautions and responsibilities).

13 All employers are required to provide adequate and appropriate equipment, facilities and personnel to enable first aid to be given to employees and others if they become ill or injured in the salon.

14 Suitably placed first aid box.
- ➤ Appointed person to take charge of first aid arrangements.

15 Infection is the invasion of the body by disease-causing micro-organisms such as bacteria, viruses, fungi and protozoa.
Infestation is the invasion of the body by animal parasites such as lice, worms and flukes. They may live in or on the body.

16 Bacteria multiply by dividing into two: this is known as binary fission.
Viruses multiply by invading a host cell causing it to make copies of the virus, which eventually destroys the host cell releasing hundreds of new viruses.

17 See pages 34–38.

18 Natural active immunity is obtained when a person comes into contact with a particular microbe and produces antibodies to repel and control it. These antibodies remain in the body to control any future infection.

19 a) Artificial active immunity can be provided by the use of vaccines. These are prepared from altered forms of the organism. They are introduced into the body, which reacts by forming antibodies.

b) Artificial passive immunity is provided by transferring antibodies from another person who has recovered from the disease.

20
- ➤ through broken or damaged skin
- ➤ through orifices
- ➤ through eyes and ears
- ➤ into hair follicles
- ➤ into the bloodstream by blood-sucking insects and lice.

See page 32 for full details.

21
- ➤ by droplet infection
- ➤ handling contaminated articles
- ➤ from dirty surfaces or dusty atmospheres
- ➤ from faeces or urine if hands are not washed thoroughly after using the toilet
- ➤ contaminated food
- ➤ contact with animals
- ➤ touching others
- ➤ through blood-sucking insects
- ➤ by contact with contaminated blood.

22 Hepatitis B and HIV are transmitted via body fluids or blood contact. May be transmitted by blood transfusion, sharing needles or any way by which blood or body fluids pass from an infected person to the recipient.

23 Ectoparasites live outside the host, e.g. lice, fleas and itch mites.
Endoparasites live inside the host, e.g. tapeworms, threadworms, roundworms or flukes.

24 See pages 40–41.

Appendix: Terminology of surfaces and structures

It is important to be familiar with the terms used to describe surfaces of the body in the anatomical position, and the position of structures relative to each other. These are shown in the following figure and described in the table overleaf.

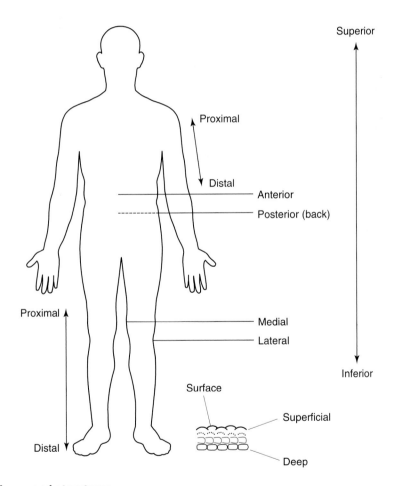

Position of surfaces and structures.

Terminology of surfaces and structures

Anterior or ventral	a surface that faces forwards; a structure that is further forwards than another
Posterior or dorsal	a surface that faces backwards; a structure that is further back than another
Medial	a surface or structure that is nearer to the mid-line than another
Lateral	a surface or structure that is further away from the mid-line than another
Proximal	a structure that is towards the root or origin, i.e. nearer the trunk
Distal	a structure that is further away from the root or origin, i.e. further away from the trunk
Superficial	a structure that is nearer the surface than others
Deep	a structure that lies beneath others, i.e. is further from the surface
Superior	a structure higher than others, i.e. nearer the head
Inferior	a structure lower than others, i.e. nearer the foot

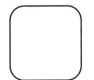

Glossary

Acid mantle a mixture of sweat and sebum that forms a coating on the skin. It is acidic with a pH of around 4.5–6; this protects the skin from infection, as it discourages the growth of micro-organisms

Adhesions fibrous tissue strands which join two surfaces that are normally separate. They form as a result of inflammation

Alveoli the air sacs of the lungs

Aponeurosis a flat sheet of connective tissue, which attaches muscles along the length of bones

Cancellous bone spongy inner mass of bone

Compact bone hard outer layer of bone

Connective tissue many different types of tissue that connect and hold other tissues together (see page 52)

Contra-action a condition that develops during the treatment, which means

stopping the treatment and taking the appropriate action

Contra-indication a condition that, if present, means that the treatment cannot be carried out

Cytoplasm jelly-like substance within a cell membrane

Desquamation the removal of the dry, scaly surface cells of the stratum corneum of the skin

Epithelium/epithelial tissue layers of cells that form the covering (skin) and linings of the body (mouth, digestive tract)

Erythema reddening of the skin produced by dilation of the blood vessels and an increase in blood flow

Exudate fluid seeping into the tissues from the blood vessels

Fasciculii muscle bundles

Homeostasis the body's inner balanced state

Hyaline cartilage a hard connective tissue that covers

the ends of bones: it reduces friction at the joints

Hygiene the precautions and procedures necessary for maintaining health and preventing the spread of disease

Hygiene requirements the hygiene standards specified by an organisation or laid down by law

Hyperaemia increase in blood flow to an area

Keratin a protein found in the skin cells that protects the skin from injury, from invasion by micro-organisms and also makes the skin waterproof

Melanin pigment found in the skin that protects against UVL rays and gives brown colour to the skin

Melanocytes cells in the skin that produce melanin

Metabolites the waste products of metabolism

Mitosis the process of cell division into two identical cells

Muscle hypertension greater than normal degree of tension in muscles

Muscle tone slight degree of tension always present in muscles, enabling them to react quickly to stimuli

Neural referring to the nervous system

Nucleus controls the activities of the cell and contains DNA

Oedema swelling of the tissues caused by an excess of tissue fluid

Organelles mini-organs that carry out the functions of a cell

Palpation the examination of the tissues through touch and feeling

Periosteum tough fibrous tissue that covers bones into which the tendons of attachment blend

Plasma proteins the protein substances suspended in the plasma of the blood, such as fibrinogen, albumin and globulin

Sensory receptors sensory nerve endings that relay sensations to the brain and spinal cord

Stasis an area of stagnation due to poor circulation

Synapse a connection between two neurones or between a neurone and its muscle fibre

Tendons tough cord-like structures of connective tissue, which attach muscles to bones

Tension nodules areas within a muscle where fibres show abnormal increase in tone

Trauma injury or damage to a part

Treatment plan the stages that you intend to follow when treating the client. It will include the aims of the treatment, the areas to be treated, the type of treatment, the timing and cost, contra-indications, any previous contra-actions, evaluation of treatment and feedback, home advice, client signature

Trigger points areas of extreme pain within the tissues, which may radiate around the area *or* may refer pain to an area some distance away

Vasoconstriction constriction of the blood vessels: the lumen becomes smaller

Vasodilation dilation of blood vessels: the lumen becomes larger

Workplace legislation all the laws and regulations governing all the activities in the workplace

Index